KETO ISLAND GIRL

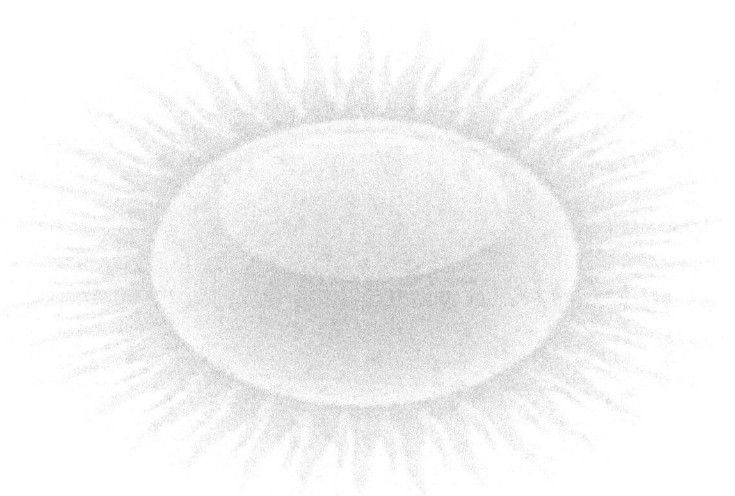

Living Healthy
Being Healthy

Copyright

November 4, 2015, by G J H

Bibliography

The Entering Wedge Society of America (1946). The Entering Wedge. The Genesis of Diet and Health.

.com (1900-2023). Brain activity and sleep. *Internet.*

.com (1900-2023). Food Values, minerals, pH, vitamins. *Internet.*

Table of Content

GJH i

PREFACE

How difficult is it to be healthy and maintain it in a fast pace world such as this? Sometimes, all it takes is a simple lifestyle, doing the things that you are already aware of; and that you know will benefit you positively.

The everyday things we can do, which is what the

book, "KETO ISLAND GIRL Living Healthy Being Healthy" is about, is recommended for both male and female, young and old, rich and poor. Here you will find the secrets to healthy living, so that if you are not yet sick you can maintain your health. But if you do become ill, you can work towards turning things around to become well again. To fully benefit and actually make the connection with what is most basic to achieve and maintain good health, you must not only read, but also put what you have read into practice. Our bodies are beautifully and wonderfully made, and it is not that difficult to be in good health. So if you want to live the way you were created to live, which is "……that thou mayest prosper and be in health, even as thy soul prospereth," 3 John 1:2 KJV, then pay attention to what you read here. All Bible verses are taken from the King James Version (KJV).

INTRODUCTION

The title portion "Living Healthy Being Healthy" was chosen because most of us came into this world as healthy babies, however, we may or may not have been able to maintain that status, depending either on how our parents took care of us initially, or because of the way we took care of ourselves thereafter. For one reason or the other we loose our health. We become sick because of a particular circumstance. But because of our nature, if we know what to do and were able to make the right changes, we could eventually overcome our illnesses, thus regaining our health. We are wonderfully made. The Bible says, "I will praise thee; for I am fearfully and wonderfully made: marvelous are thy works; and that my soul knoweth right well," Psalm 139:14 KJV. The process of living healthily is what can pose the most problems, since maintaining it takes some form of commitment. This written project is designed to bring us to this awareness. So that if at present we are not sick, we will be able to avoid getting sick. But, if we are or become ill, it can be quickly reversed so that healthy living can be achieved once again.

And now, here is an account of how I, an island girl went from a state of well being, to suddenly becoming severely ill, then back to being healthy again, without the help of a physician.

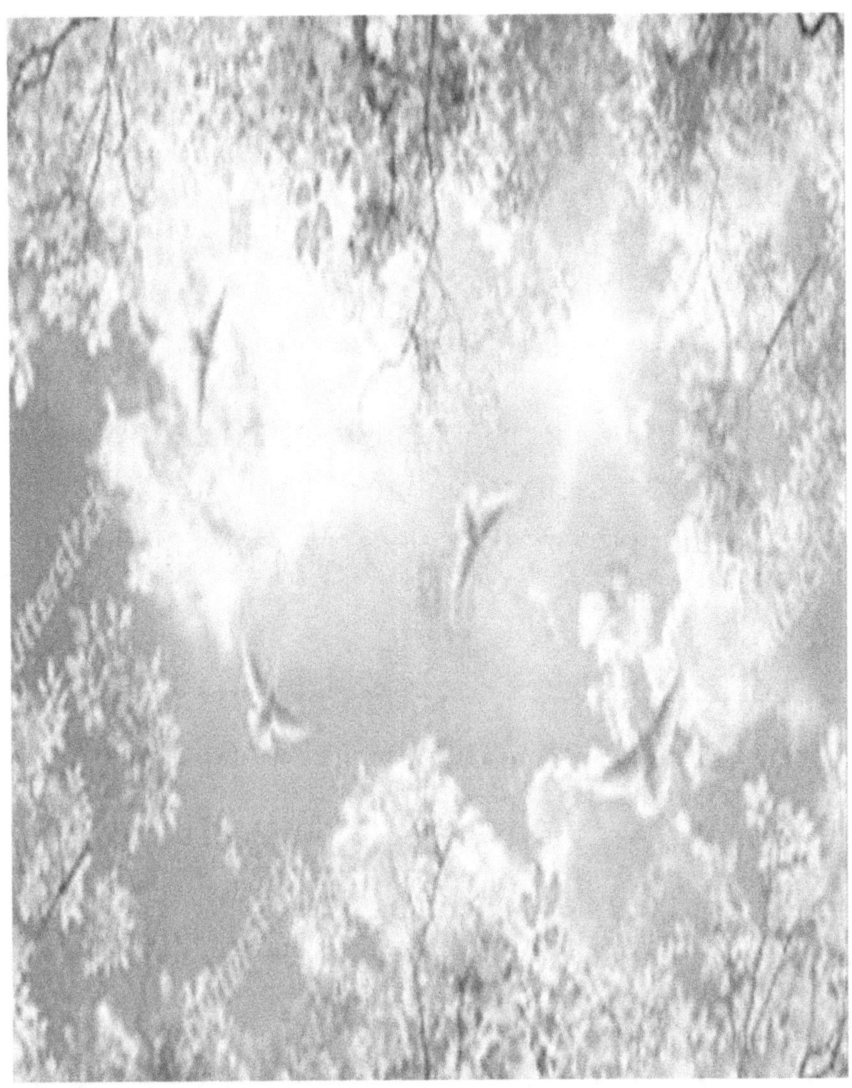

A Day in the Sun

I knew nothing else but being healthy.

GJH vi

PART ONE::: My initial lifestyle: the physical.

Words of Wisdom

"A fit, healthy body – that is the best fashion statement."

---Jess Scott

"When health is absent, wisdom cannot reveal itself, art cannot manifest, strenght cannot fight, wealth becomes useless, and intelligence cannot be applied."

---Heroplilus

"I'd rather have my health than silver and gold."

---Grace J Habib

"Eat breakfast as a king, lunch as a prince and dinner as a pauper. Better yet, eat only two meals daily: breakfast and dinner."

---Grace J Habib

Hello, my name is Grace. Let me tell you about my life story, about how I first became sick, and then about how I regained my health. It is a unique story. And because I have an awareness of the fact that there are so many illnesses in the world today, which really can be avoided, I now feel compelled to share this account. You see, once upon a time I always felt sound, then suddenly, my well being got away from me. But I was finally able to regain it with a little determination and without the help of a doctor. I began to realize, that initially what came so naturally, was the only simple way to begin to improve on a situation that had gone so horribly wrong. Then, after much effort, I soon began to regain that which I had lost. And now I aim to maintain my health on a daily basis. The facts pertaining to everyday living are all here, and are woven in such a manner as to pull you in, so that you can almost experience it too. And now, here is a picture of my life in my youth. So come along and begin to take this journey with me.

I grew up on an island in the sun. It was a very small carribean island, where practically everybody, and especially in neighborhoods, knew everyone else. The people were family oriented and there was much togetherness amongst the neighbors, therefore people shared with each other. I remember the holiday seasons, when families would visit each other, going to one another's homes and sharing whatever there was to eat. Along with this, there was lots of conversation and good laughter. It was just plain simple fun. There was love and togetherness in my family. The house that I grew up in was situated in what one might call country, because it was about four miles away from the island's city area, quite secluded and one of the only places on the island that did not have a beach. The house was built on ten acres of land, and on the land, my family planted many different fruit trees. Let me name a few of those tropical fruits. There were mangoes, plums, cane, coconuts, keneps, cherries, cocoa, coffee, sapodillas, sea grapes, oranges, and pomorac, guava, grapefruits, mandarine, tangerine, lemons, limes, custard apple, guayabana, cimates and avocado to name a few, and the list goes on and on. These are just some of the fruit trees that were on the land. There were many more; but just to name this many, and to mention that there were even more, would give you an idea of what it was like, to have all of this at my disposal year round. It was either this friut or that, all in their own season. I could just pick and eat them vined ripe straight from off the tree. Trust me, every day was a fun

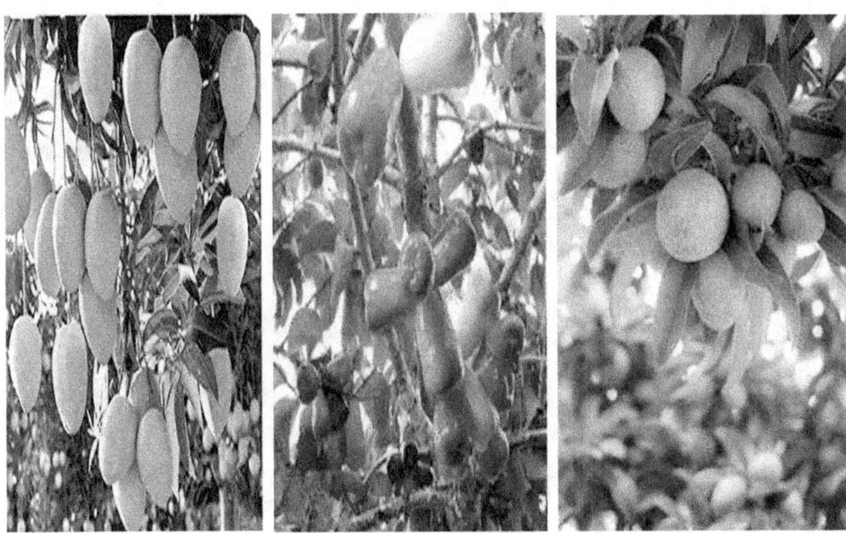

Mangoe, Pomerac and Sapodilla Fruit Trees

day. Just to be able to go to any fruit tree of my choice, and as long as that fruit was ripe, I could reach up and pick it off of the tree and eat. I did not have to go to the store and purchase force riped fruit when I wanted a particular fruit. Whatever I wanted I could just pick and eat. Literally, I could just reach my hand up to that vined riped fruit, ripened on the tree in the sun, pick it and eat. This to me was healthy living.

Another area of organic eating besides vined ripe

fruits was from the planting of our own vegetables. These were fertilized naturally using

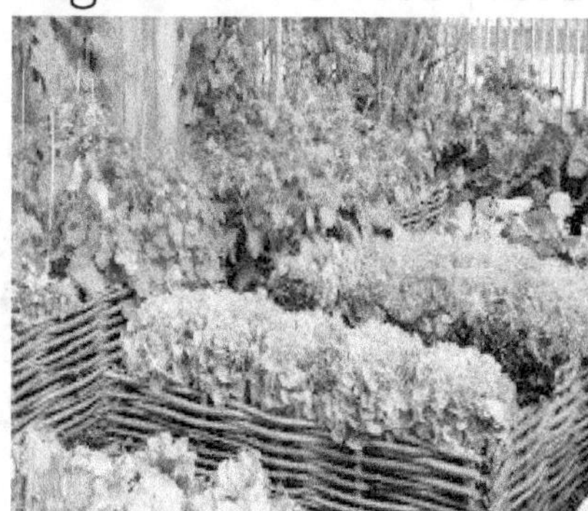
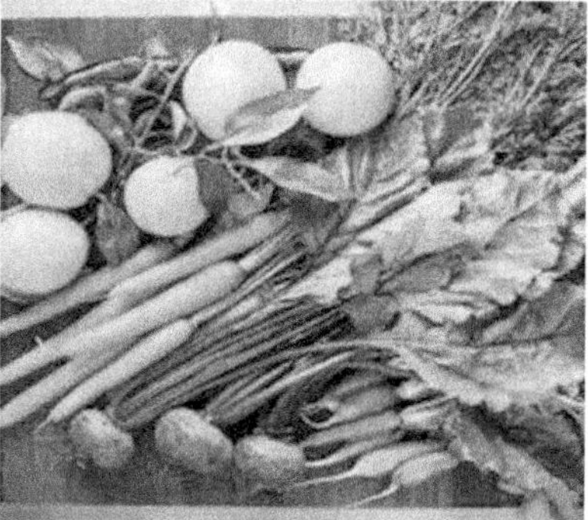

Home Grown Fruits and Vegetables

mainly cow patties. There were no artificial fertilizers or sprays used in planting. Besides that, there were no chemicals in the soil or in the water. The rains came often, and the water coming through the taps (faucets) from the reservoir was not treated with lots of chemicals.

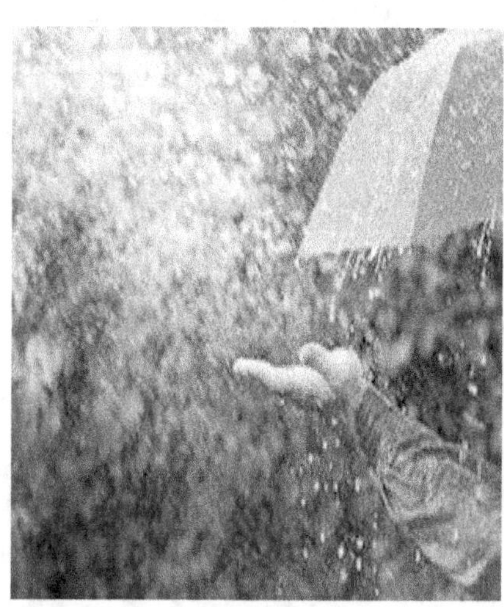
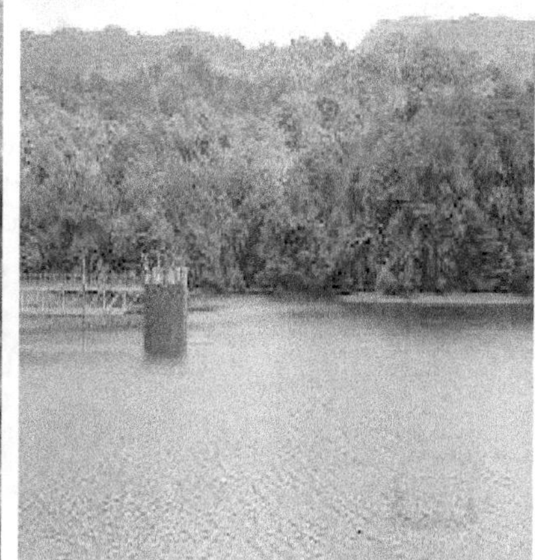

The Rainy Season: The Reservoir

Both fruits and vegetables were therefore organic, and no one feared for their safety in eating them because these were mostly home grown. They were watered from the rain having no chemtrail residue, and hosed with water from the faucet flowing from the reservoir with not many chemicals, if any at all in it.

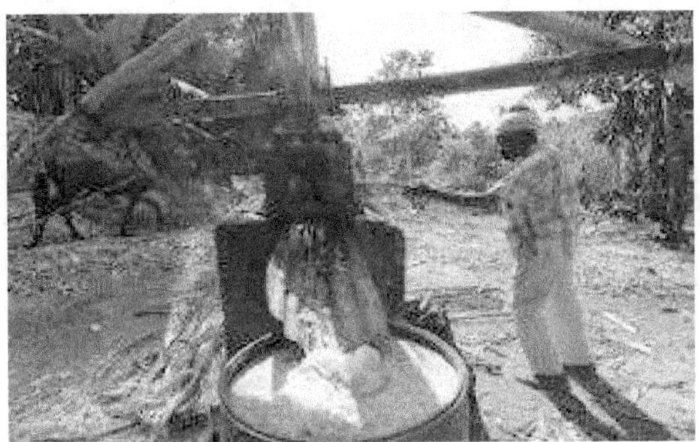

Sugar Cane and Old fashion Sugar Mill

The sugar was locally made on the island. And by using our own home-grown cane, we could make an even purer form of brown sugar called wet sugar. There was also another method of processing cane juice to form a type of sweetener called molasses. Processed, granulated and confection sugar were hardly used. But in the case of making and beautifying wedding cakes and making candies, they were used. This greatly lessened the chances of the nation becoming diabetic. I am not saying that people never got sick with these and other diseases, but what I am saying is that it was more the norm for people to maintain themselves in a more desirable manner.

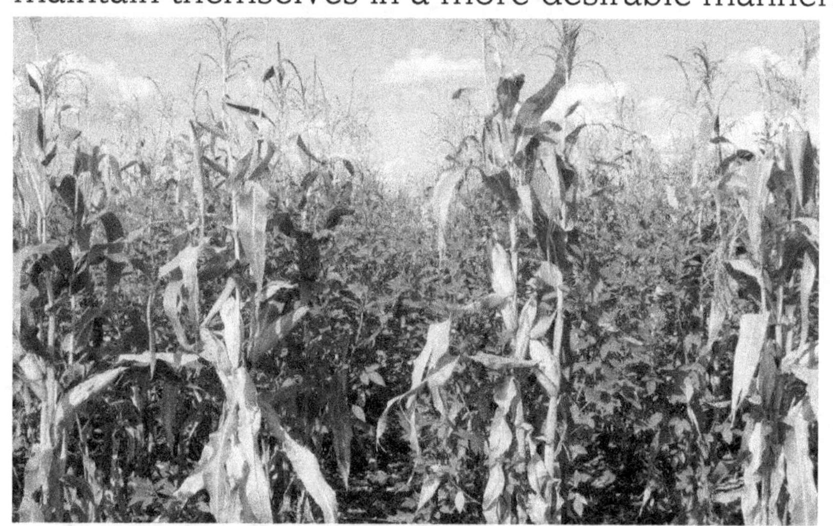

Intercropping Maize with Pigeon Peas

Some foods were grown seasonally. Here, I am speaking of things like corn and pigeon peas. At a certain time of the year, the island's natives, those of us who were interested in planting, grew our own corn and peas. The land was first prepared and dugged. Then corn and pigeon peas, after first being treated to repel bugs were placed in the same hole opposite to each other in the ground. They grew, they blossomed, and in time they were harvested. No seed was modified, and when these were picked, all original nutrients were maintained in them. When you ate them, you were eating a good meal, and whatever was not harvested immediately when they were green and ripened, could, after they became dry, be kept as long as necessary and eaten at a later date. Nothing had to be thrown away. Nothing had to be wasted. There was enough for the present, and enough that could be preserved for future use. There was no need to use chemicals to preserve them. The nutritional value of these produce were preserved when dried, even up until the following season, depending on how

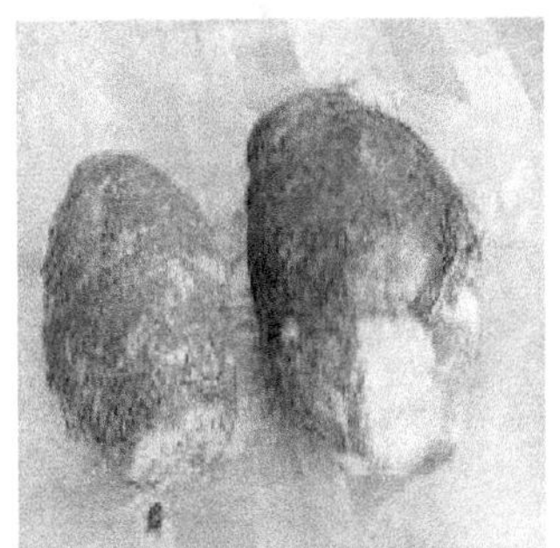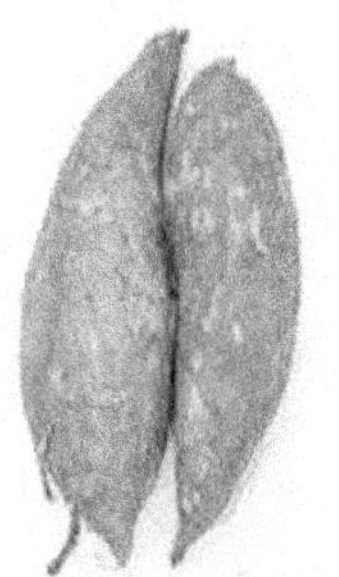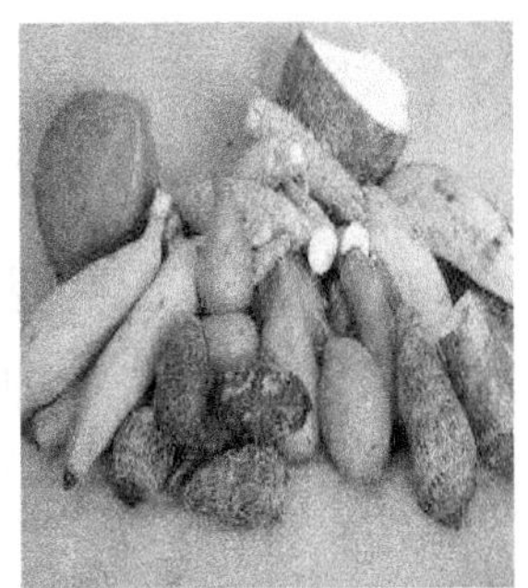

Ground Provision

they were stored for the future. There was also year-round planting of ground provision such as dasheen (malanga), tania, yam, cassava, and sweet potatoes. You may or may not know what some of these root tubers are. However, in some foreign countries, you can find them in the produce section of some supermarkets. Just try to remember what you have seen that is not familiar to your country but imported from the Caribbean, and you will begin to get a clearer picture of what is spoken of here. These are just some of the ways that home grown foods were produced, with no chemicals involved; but by just using the God-given ground, His water, and if necessary, dung from clean edible animals such as the cow and sheep as fertilizers.

And now I post a question. What are many acres of land without animals on it? They actually help to keep grass low and the land clean by grazing. Eating their fresh land grass gave me wide clear open fields of acreage to run, jump and play on, in the bright vitamin D filled sun. So much for paying to exercise at a gym. And why did I have to do that, when I had all the exercise I needed by walking, jumping, running, and climbing trees on vast wide-open land. So there, I could maintain strong muscles. I could burn off calories with all that exercise. That was so much fun so that it didn't even feel like doing a workout. It just felt like another day in paradise. And for the animals, it was the same. I saw how the goat kids skipped. They too were happy. Their moms and dads grazed to their hearts desire.

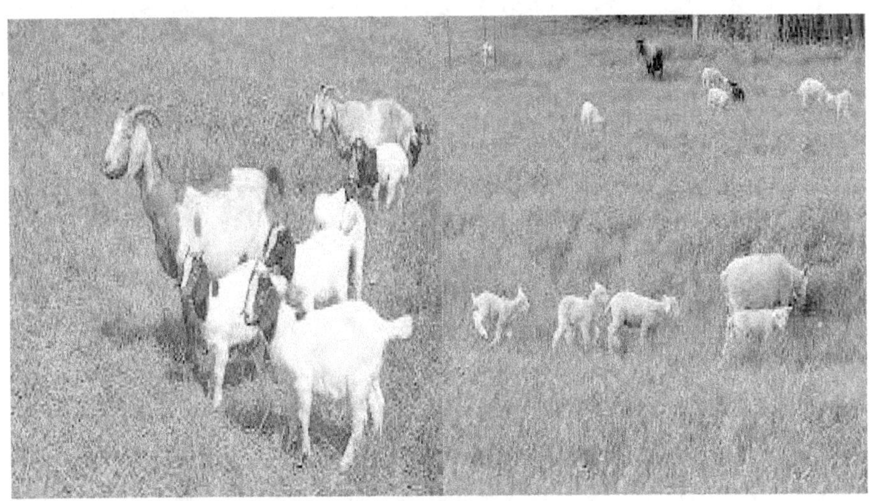

Goats with Their Kids and Sheep with Their Lambs.

The sheep and lambs did their own thing too. And the cows mooed and grazed as they were moved from one part of the land to the next from their tied positon. Some animals had to be tied to keep them from straying onto the neighbours land. The chicken, ducks, guinea birds and turkeys shuffeled in and out of fallen dried leaves, without a care in the world. The pigs were kept in pens, and I felt badly that they had to be penned up. But their was one pig called Choicey who was the exception. She was the prized pig: the cream of the crop, everyone's favorite. We all loved her. I will tell you a little more about Choicey later.

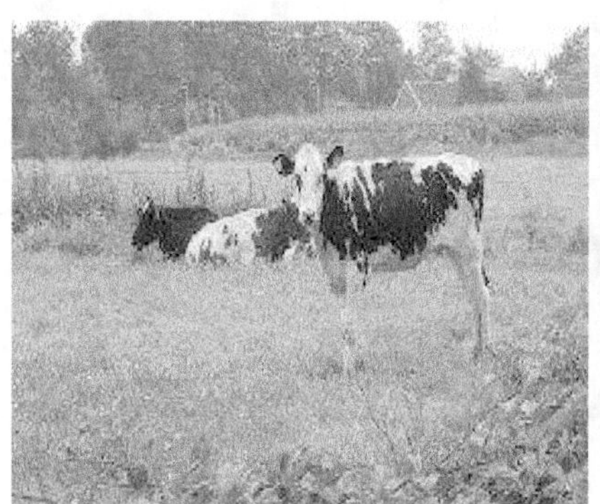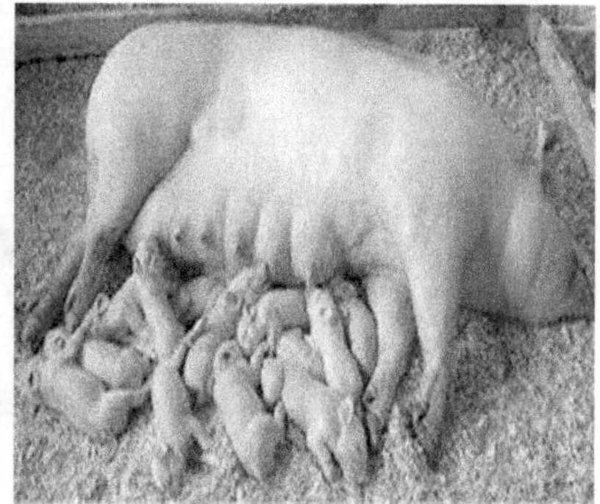

Cows and Pigs

The doves flew here and there, but always came home in the evening to sleep. The rabbits seemed happy in their cages. The dogs did their job to bark and keep trouble at bay for the family. And the cats, well, they meowed, stretched, ran in and out of the house, rubbed against your legs, and looked at you in such a way behaving as if you owed them something.

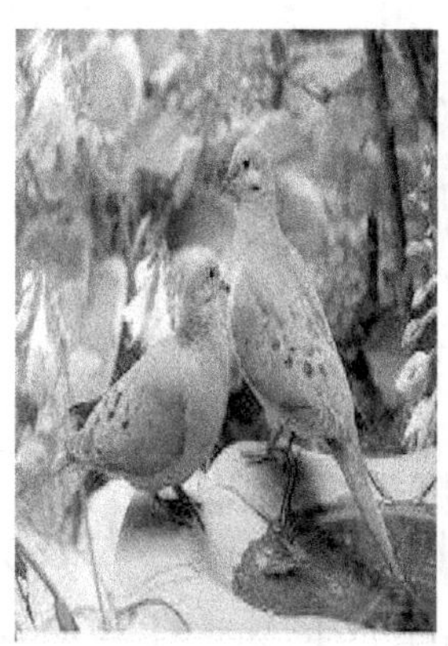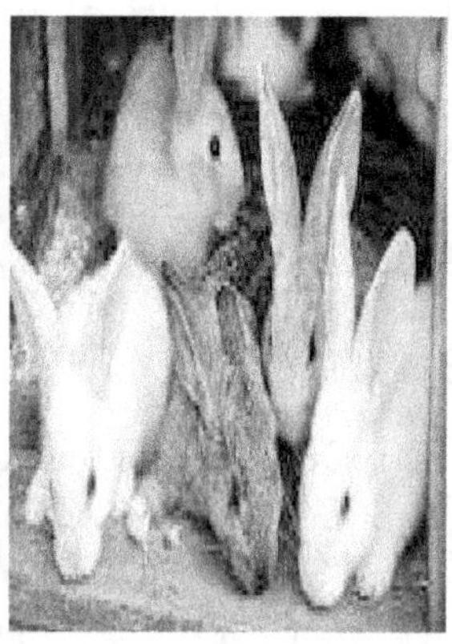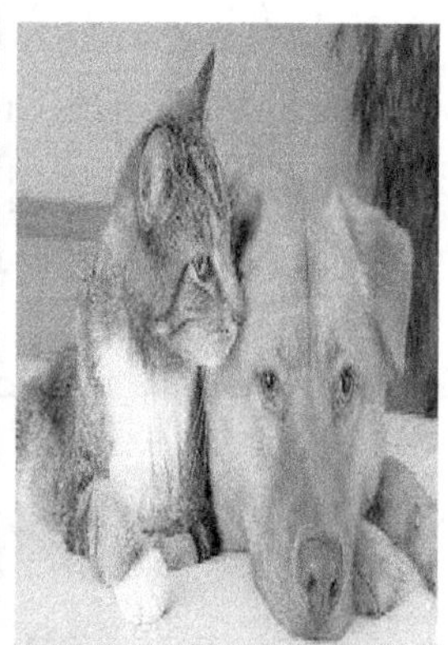

Dove/Pigeons, Rabbits, Loving Cat and Dog

You might be wondering why I have taken the

time to mention all these animals. Well, the reason is twofold. The first reason is because we had them, and the second reason is that we were able to interact with them as if they were part of the family. So many different animals produced a calm and peaceful atmosphere, made depression to be a thing unknown, and created much happier surroundings. As the saying goes, "A dog is a man's best friend." But guess what, all the other animals were likewise to me as friends. They were not troublesome but gave a unique kind of flare to nature itself. They could not speak, so I could love them without worrying about whether they were genuine, or if they would turn around and gossip about me behind my back. Therefore, there was no mistrust between them and me. They were my friends.

The result of having these animals as friends was twofold. The first is that they were instrumental in putting and keeping me in a mentally calm state, because of the peaceful atmosphere which they created. The fact of the matter is that a healthy mental state is just as important, or maybe even more so than your healthy physical state. And because of this, I really loved being around them.

They were my pets. The second reason for mentioning the animals is because of the food which some of them provided. Maybe you have noticed that there is a recent trend called vegetarianism; but back then, when I was growing up on the island, people ate just about anything they wanted to. And I was no exception to this. We were all meat eaters, and this included Christians.

You might be wondering why I keep talking about food. Well, it's because that is what makes our blood. If you want good blood, then you must eat good food. And if you want a healthy life then you must have good healthy blood. After all, didn't the Bible say that "the life is in the blood." Leviticus 17:11 KJV. So, let's begin to look at the lifestyle of these animals, and see whether some of them were fit for human consumption.

The first point here, as it pertains, is how the animals lived. The second point of interest is what they ate. The animals had freedom to move up and down in fresh air and under the sun, on the many acres of land. They could go wherever they wanted to go and do whatever they wanted to do without restriction. The cows moored, and along with the sheep and goats, they walked the length and breadth of the land based on where they were tied to graze, but they were never penned up. They ate chemically untreated grass, grown on chemically untreated soil, exposed to daily sunlight, and got wet from rainwater and night dew.

So clear it is that if the soil was healthy then the grass was healthy; the water was uncontaminated, and the air fresh. Therefore, what the animals ate was also supposed to be healthy, and when we ate those animals, then we too were healthy. This also applied to birds and poultry. The way dairy, fruits and vegetables were produced, and their preparations in cooking and baking, was consequently equivalent to what we would consider today as being organic.

The pigs, however, were different. They had to be kept in stalls and were fed just about anything and everything. I could never figure out back then why whenever I ate pork, my stomach would feel nauseated. Not until I read Leviticus chapter 11 KJV and found out that the pig was unclean, and unfit for human consumption, that is when I stopped eating pork to my benefit. But even so, I still liked seeing the pigs among the other animals, as I also thought of them as pets.

Remember Choicey? I mentioned her earlier on. Now let me tell you a little more about her, and how she made everyone at home so very happy. Choicey was a fully grown very fat pig, very intelligent and very friendly. Willing to give a show whenever the opportunity arose and always had a willing audience. The simple things she did were always entertaining, only because no other

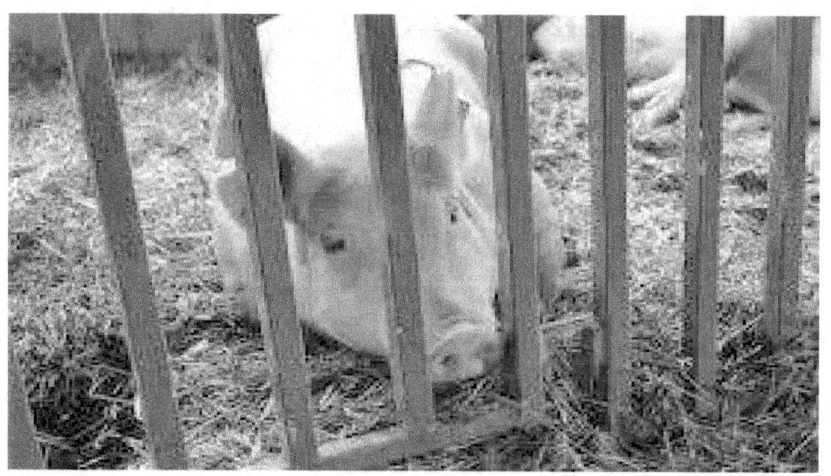

Choicey

animal did them. Now let's see what she did. Choicey would use her mouth to unlatch the door of her stall, stroll out of her stall, go to the faucet in the yard, turn it on with her mouth, drink water, take a bath and then bask in the sun for a while. Then, when she got ready and decided that she had had enough, and that it was a good time to go back home, she would then get up and stroll back to her stall at leisure. What a statement. It was like she was saying, "I am Choicey, and nobody tells me what to do." She was not only an independent thinker but also a teacher, because

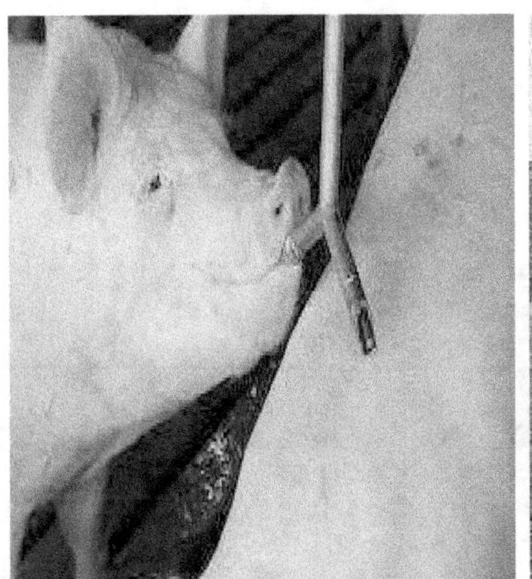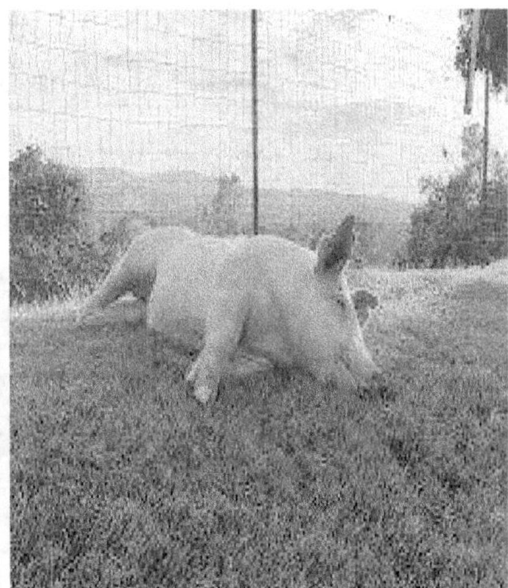

Choicey the Smart Pet

at that time, we didn't know that a pig could do these things before Choicey came along. And what she did brought us entertainment. I don't remember how she died; if she became a holiday meal or whether she died of natural causes. But she left such an impression on the minds of everyone in the entire family, so much so that even up to today, she can still be a topic of conversation among those of us who experienced her. I have a first cousin who named one of his daughters after this sow. You see, she was that special. Needless to say, he named his daughter Choicey. The pig, however, was not the only source of meat that was not good for us to eat, even though it found its way onto the dinner table. We also ate meat that was commonly known on the island as bush meat. I remember my uncles and a few of their friends hunting wild animals such as opossums, iguanas, and

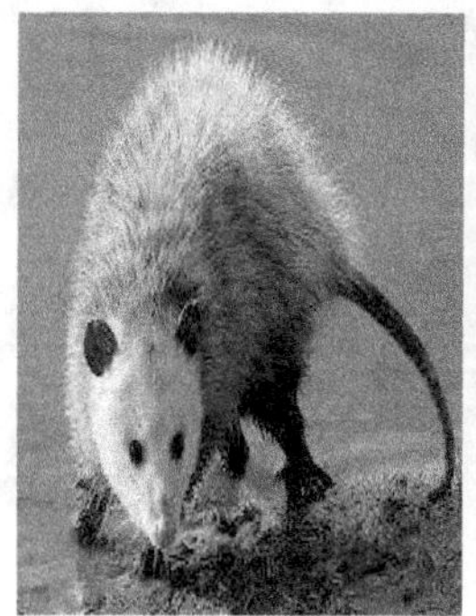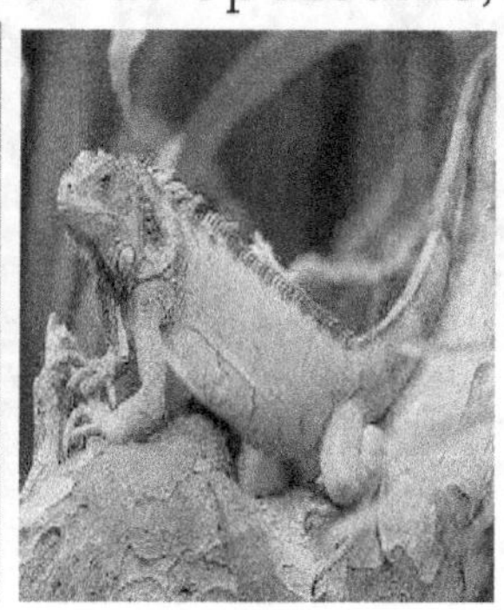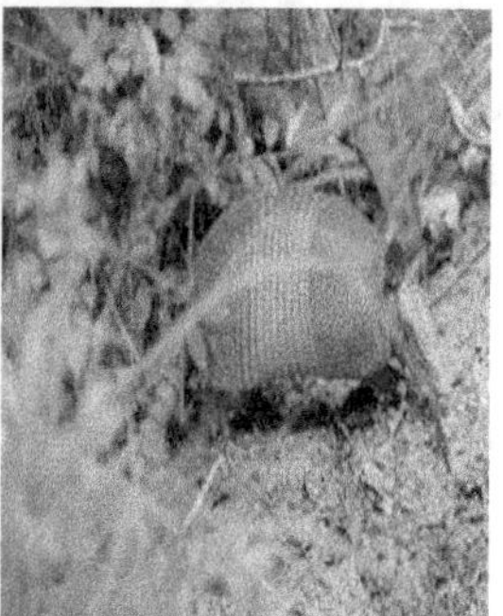

Opossum, Iguana, and Armadillo

armadillos. They caught them, seasoned, and cooked those meats with coconut milk, which made that food taste exceptionally good. Coconut milk was not the problem, but for the wild meats, oh no, we should never have eaten such things which, based on Leviticus chapter 11 KJV says we should not eat, because these are unclean meats. For example, "And the swine, though he divide the hoof, and be clovenfooted, yet he cheweth not the cud; he is unclean to you," Leviticus 11:7 KJV. But the Most High was good to us. He never allowed us to get sick because back then, we didn't know any better.

And then there were animals that came from the ocean and some of them were also unclean. Not good for human consumption. These were mainly sharks and turtles, and there was also something that resembled sea cockroaches and barnacles that lived, attaching themselves to ocean rocks. My grandmother made a sort of tea with them, but I can't remember ever drinking that tea. I did eat shark and turtle though, which tasted really good, but after eating two pieces of turtle, I couldn't eat a third piece, because I would begin to feel nauseated. This was a big red flag to tell me to put the brakes on, and not continue to eat this thing, since it was obviously not good for me to consume. Today I no longer eat these unclean meats. Thank you Most High. You have been so good to me!

So as you can see, our flesh foods whether coming from the land or sea were divided into two group (1) clean and (2) unclean, but somehow irregardless of what we ate, besides a little nausea, overall I didn't really get sick. And

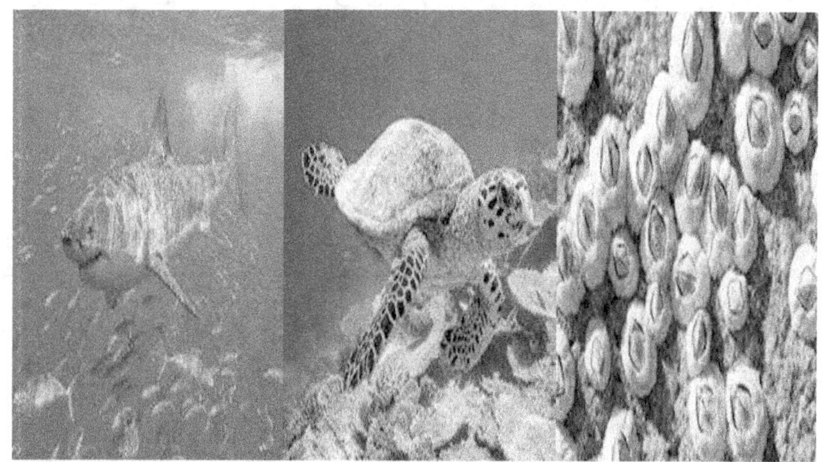

Unlean Fish: Shark, Turtle and Barnacles

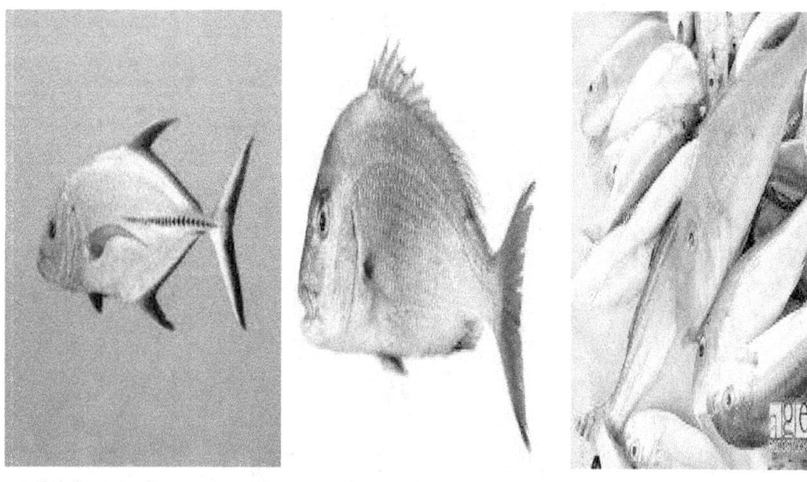

Edible Fish with Fins and Scales

GJH 19

once I felt nauseated, I stopped eating whatever was responsible for causing this discomfort. It took a while, but since then I began transitioning into becoming a vegetarian, then into becoming a vegan: which is a much more wholesome way of eating: something I have maintained doing, even up to today.

The atmosphere, the enviroment and the surroundings on this island all blended together, creating an unsurpassed calm enjoyed by all. But to say that there was never anything negative, referring to the usual country pest such as things like ants, cockroaches, mice and snakes would be a lie. They too were there, yet, with its own share of difficulties, swiftly gotten rid of. However, not withstanding any discomfort they brought, even the giant snails slowly clawling across the yard at midday in the hot sun, had their own way of telling a story, that the land was home to all: a credit to Yahuveh's glory!

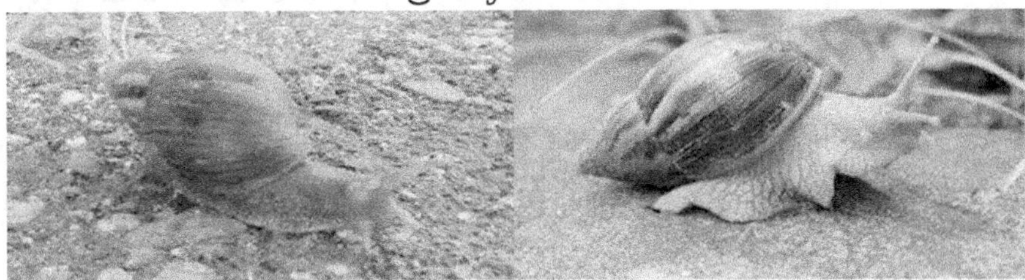

The Happy Snails

PART TWO::: The Psychological

So far, I have dealt with the physical aspect of growing up on the islands. But what is the physical without the psychological? How much more important is the mental aspect of the issue, and this was the dealings of it. Here everyone was taught the principle that if what you were thinking or doing would be harmful to you or to others, then it was not the thing to be doing. Sad to say though, many people failed to live by this principle. Some people used witchcraft (obeah) against others to succeed financially, or to hinder other people's progress, and sexual abuse even within the family could not be discounted off. It happened! And because of witchcraft and incest, lives were ruined permanently. On the other hand, if it was okay to do the thing that you were thinking of doing, then yes, you could go ahead and do it, but not overdo

"Too much of one thing is good for nothing."

GJH 21

it. There is an old saying on the island that goes like this; "Too much of one thing is good for nothing." And just knowing what we should or should not have been doing, and being taught right from wrong in different areas of life, made all the difference not just fot the culture but also for the welfare of the world.

Parental guidance was a very strong aspect as part of the island's culture. And when I say parental guidance, I am talking about the fact that it took a community to raise a child. For instance, culturally, certain things were obviously taught in the home; things that were familiar, not only to one family but to the typical family across board. Teaching children right from wrong, to love Yahuveh and His Son Yahushua HaMashiach, and to go to church weekly whether Sabbath keeper or Sunday keeper; is how it was done, and I don't think any one family was lacking in this area. The island was mainly Catholic, but gradually Seventh Day Adventism and other Sabbath keeping religions claimed their place on the island, along with a few heathen religions, one such among others being hinduism. If anyone, whether adult or child, went against the norm to choose a negative persuasion, and blatantly executed it, then it was of their own choosing, and their actions went against community standards. Needless to say, if it was a matter serious enough and against the law, then the police would get involved and as long as it could be proven, justice would be served. There is an old adage that goes like this, "It takes a village to raise a child."

"It takes a village

to raise a child."

How true in this case, because if anyone saw me doing something that they thought I should not be doing, it would be reported to my elders at home, and if that report was found to be true, then I would be punished for it. It was expected that children would obey their elders both in and out of the home to do right. It was also expected that of the two opposing lifestyles, either good or bad, everyone would choose to be good. But it was not so. Some actually chose to do evil; ever breeding a regular source of gossip. The island was so small that practically everyone knew everyone else's business. Believe it or not, even in these modern times there was and still is no lack of noseness while living there.

A life without Fear

No one lived in fear or was overanxious on this island. What a peaceful environment surrounded by oceans and such cool breeze, with sandy

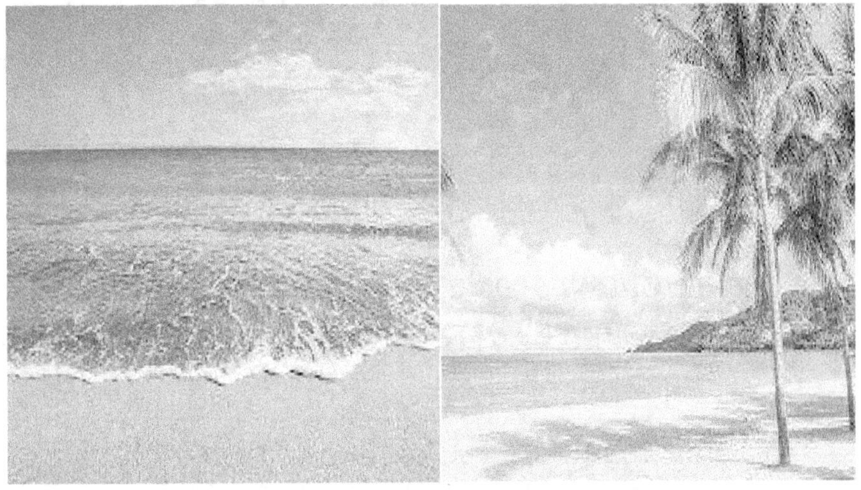

Sandy Shores and Coconut Trees

shores and coconut trees. People could be out at anytime day or night, and no one would get harmed. Murders and rapes were basically nil. I cannot remember even one murder committed on that small island when I lived there.

You could just be outside enjoying the moonlight. And what bright and calming moonlight; so bright compared with the sun. Sometimes at night when

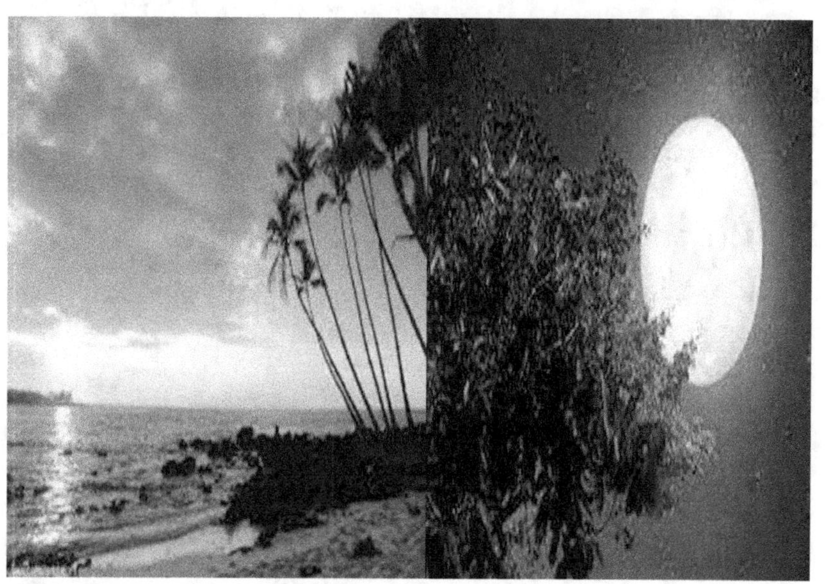

Such Beautiful Moonlight

everyone was asleep, I would get out of bed, and go sit in the yard by myself just to enjoy serenity and the beauty of the moon. I had no fear of being alone. Those nights were so bright. People on the island were taught from their youth to refuse the evil and choose the good. And this is exactly how it was. So, because of high moral standards, the island was peaceful and quiet. No one lived in fear of anything or anyone else.

Occasionally from time to time I would hear

about a child disrespecting their parents, but it was very rear. The community was like one big family. And even when people did not know one another, when they did meet each other for the first time, it was so easy to connect because of the prevailing atmosphere. These island people had a connection because there was a common denominator among us of choosing what was good, and avoiding that which was not. For a better understanding and to get a broader picture of the prevailing lifestyle here, let me present a few examples. Here are three.

Example number one:- I was thought that while walking on the road, a good practice was to say good morning, good afternoon, good evening and good night to whomever I met. To do this was to show respect for that person. I never knew back then why it was so important to treat strangers like this until I read this text in the Bible which says, "Let brotherly love continue. Be not forgetful to entertain strangers, for thereby some have entertained angels unawares." Hebrew13:1-3 KJV.

" *Let brotherly love continue. Be not forgetful to entertain strangers, for thereby some have entertained angels unawares, Hebrews 13:1-3 KJV.*

Example number two :- There was once a hurricane on the island, and practically all the the surrounding houses were blown down, but the house in which I grew up was untouched. It stood up unaffected by the winds. And both during the storms, when people's houses were blowing in

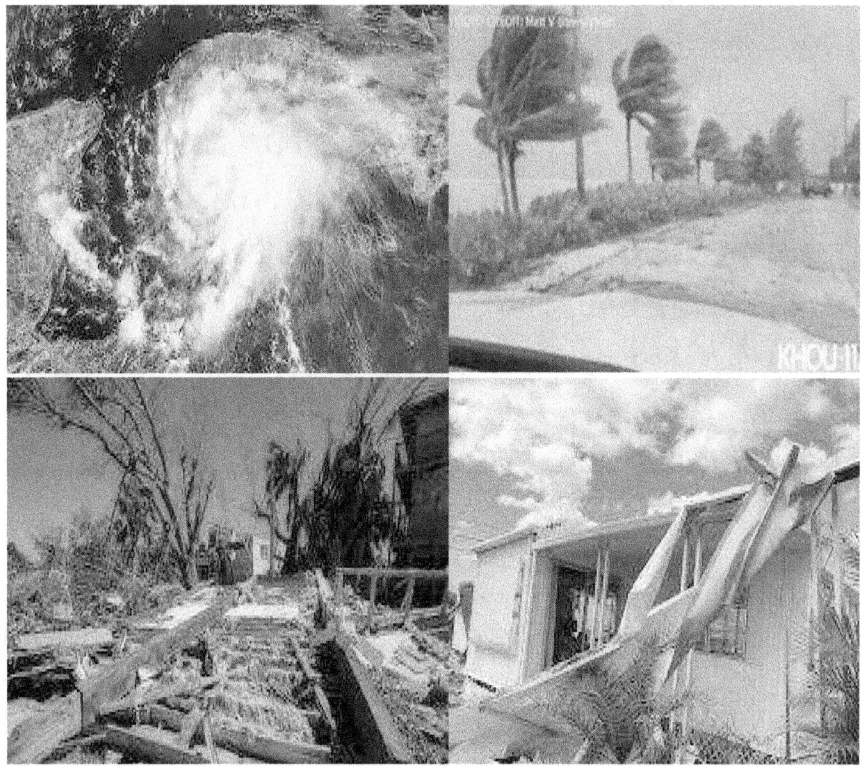

Hurricane Winds and Destruction

the winds and when the hurricane was over, and the search for survivors began, people who lost their houses either came or were brought to our home. As a matter-of-fact, they started running up to the house during the torm. It literally became a shelter and hospital. The villagers just knew that the arms of my family would be willingly opened to help them. And so it was. We helped them until they were able to get back on their feet.

Example number three :- Every time I think of this event it sort of makes me sad, and now I will tell you what happened. I was so young at the time, when I saw a young man who for one reason or the other was put out of his house. He came to my folks and asked them to take him in, but they refused. I never understood why they did that at the time, because they were always so accommodating. But when I look back on it, the only thing I could think about of why they made that decision, was that there were innocent girls living in the house, and they didn't want anyone to come in and take advantage of us. You see, virtue was a very important aspect of life. It was something that was taught to me; therefore, I was able to pass it on to my children, and now they will be able to pass it on to their children. Don't get me wrong now. Stuff happened along the way. But at least they did what they were supposed to do by teaching us

GJH **29**

how important it was to respect our virtue.

Life on the island was always very calm, no hustle and bustle; one today two tomorrow. Everyday was just another day in paradise. This applied to every area including school and the working world. Our schedule was pretty much the same every day. Things remained pretty much unchanged. Everyday brought a typical day. School began at 9.00 AM in the morning and ended at 3.00 PM in the afternoon. In many cases, if there was something extra to be done, time for that would be squeezed in during the school day. Staying over in the afternoon was pretty much discouraged. When it was time to go home, it was time to go home. Work began at 8:00 AM and ended at 4:00 PM, except when there was a variation in the time schedule. For instance, in the case of working extra hours when an election was coming up, if you worked in the Election Department of the civil service like I did.

Another example would be working at the hospital which required working second or third shift. There was only one hospital and no nursing homes at that time on the island. Most people took care of the elderly and sick at home, except in extreme cases when someone needed to be taken to the hospital. And those who worked off shifts obviously lost sleep.

There were elementary schools in various villages and districts, so students usually walked to and from school. It was a bit different with the High (secondary) schools though, since there were not many, and those were located only in certain areas of the island. Here is where most students needed a ride to go to school, but high school students who lived close to their school could walk. The benefits of walking was twofold. i- It was good exercise, and ii- By doing so, it helped the body to get tired enough so that falling asleep naturally without a sleep aid would be easier and faster. This also resulted in enough sound sleep, which rested the brain especially after doing much homework. The word insomnia was never mentioned in my hearing. I never knew that it existed, even though I am sure some people might have had that problem. By 8:00 PM, almost everyone was already in bed getting enough sleep, to wake up early the next morning to begin our daily routine. Although school was demanding, most students excelled, and this was because among other things we got such a good night's rest continually. By the way, high school was the **bomb.** I really loved it. It's the one part of my life that empatically made me happy, and if I could choose, I would do it again in a heart beat!

Those Open Houses

There is something to be said about how the houses were built which promoted good sleep. Houses were not built in such a way to prevent fresh air from coming into the rooms. Ventilation was good, and the air was fresh and clean. While we slept, for the most part, we only breathed fresh well oxygenated air. This was so since there was a lot of vegetation and next to no combustion, from the very few vehicles driven in in my neighborhood; in my neck of the woods, so to speak. If you could form a picture in your mind of what it was like on that island back then, you would even say that it was a virgin type living. Getting to bed on time and sleeping in a well-ventilated room promoted good circulation, while removing impurities from the blood. This was evident when we woke up, because our eyes would contain a sticky substance called yam-pee. It was formed from impurities continually being removed from our blood nightly, through that part of our body while we slept. Sleep quality was better than good. The air quality was great. The food quality was excellent. Exercise didn't feel like exercise. There was no added effort there. It felt normal and that was fun.

I want to be honest though and make it plain that as people aged, some of them did have health problems such as diabetes from eating too much sweet foods, hypertension because of eating spicy foods and eye problems because of diabetes or just plain old age. There were other health problems with the aged, but I didn't see many overweight people. Both young and old were strong. Most young people maintained good health in general, and even though there were exceptions, most aged people lived to a good old age.

Relaxation

Relaxation was also very important and to us pretty basic. It was a normal part of our existence. No one was forced to relax because life was not really stressful. And if those in responsible positions were stressed out in any way, many times it was not made apparent to children in the family. The grownups had a way of keeping their problems to themselves. One of the main things expected of us, was to treat our elders with respect, and do what we were told to do. If we were obedient, we remained pretty stress free and better able to live a relaxed life. Our lifestyle was what affected our mood. No effort was made to meditate. My mind was always free to drift into a dream world. I was a daydreamer. I dreamt a lot. Sometimes I would just drift into an unexpected daydream and that was so sweet. There were however, activities designed purely for recreational purposes. Some of these activities included going to the beach. I had never been to the beach by myself, it was always a group project with friends and family, enjoying a special time together. And the beaches were heavenly. They were calm and aquamarine in color. And because the sun was always shining except in the rainy season, the water was, in most cases, just quite so warm and glistening under the sun.

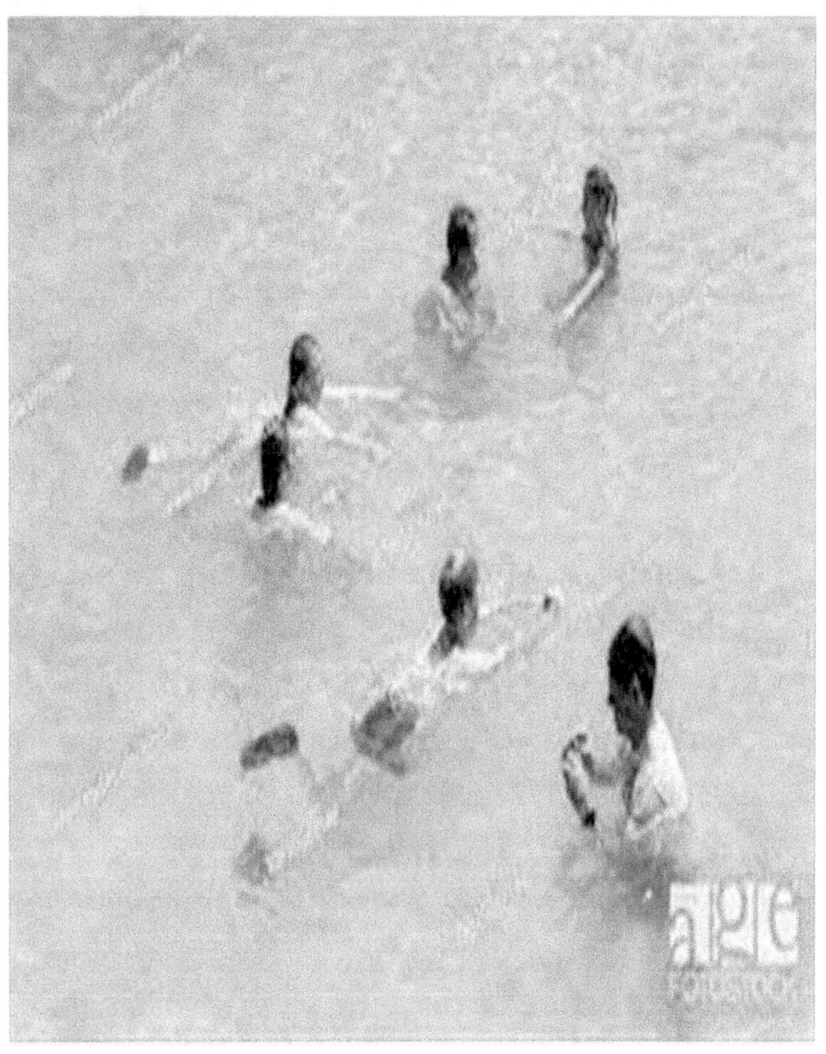

Ocean Pool Inside the Reef

On this island, there is a reef with a pool out in the inner section of the ocean, in a portion of one of the more popular beaches. But I never got an opportunity to go there in my youth. After I became an adult and revisited the island, I finally got a chance to visit the reef, and that is when I realized, what a wonder of the world I had missed while growing up. I went there in a glass bottom

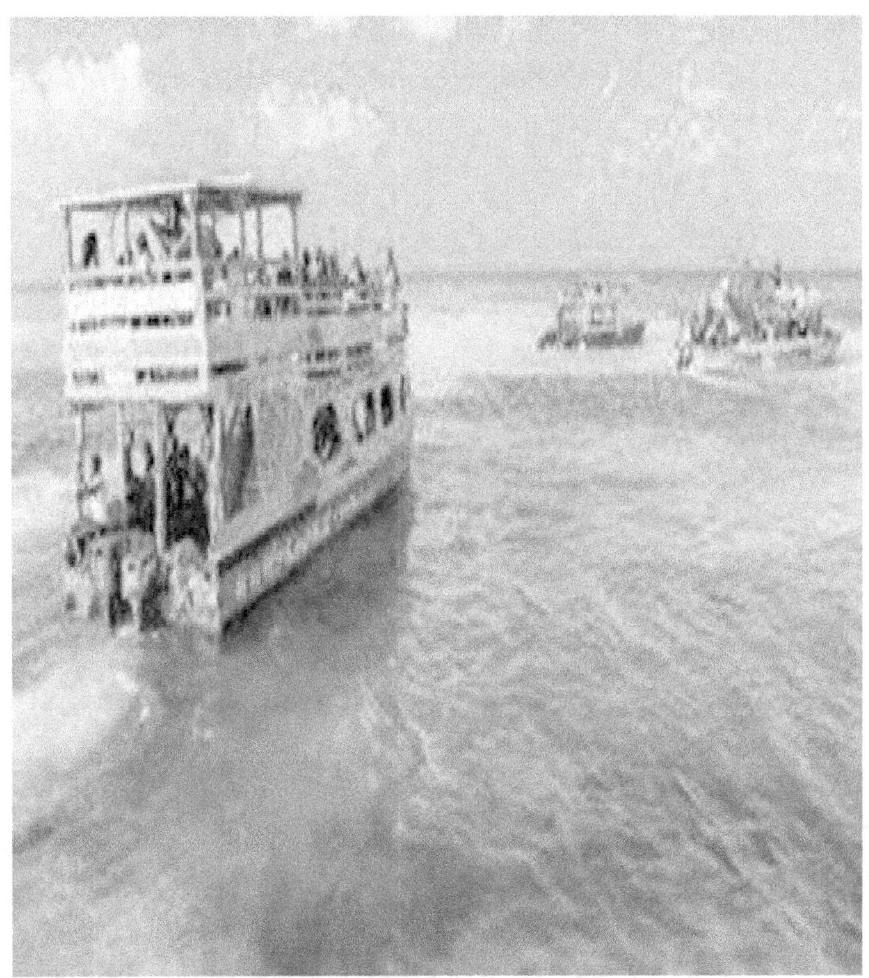

Glass Bottom Boat

boat. Beneath my feet I could see coral and all types of fishes. It was picturesque.

As I got out of that boat, I could see different

types of fishes through the shiny clear water. They swam around my feet, and I could walk amongst them. In another section of the ocean right before getting to the reef, anyone could get out and snorkel. Hence, with that experience

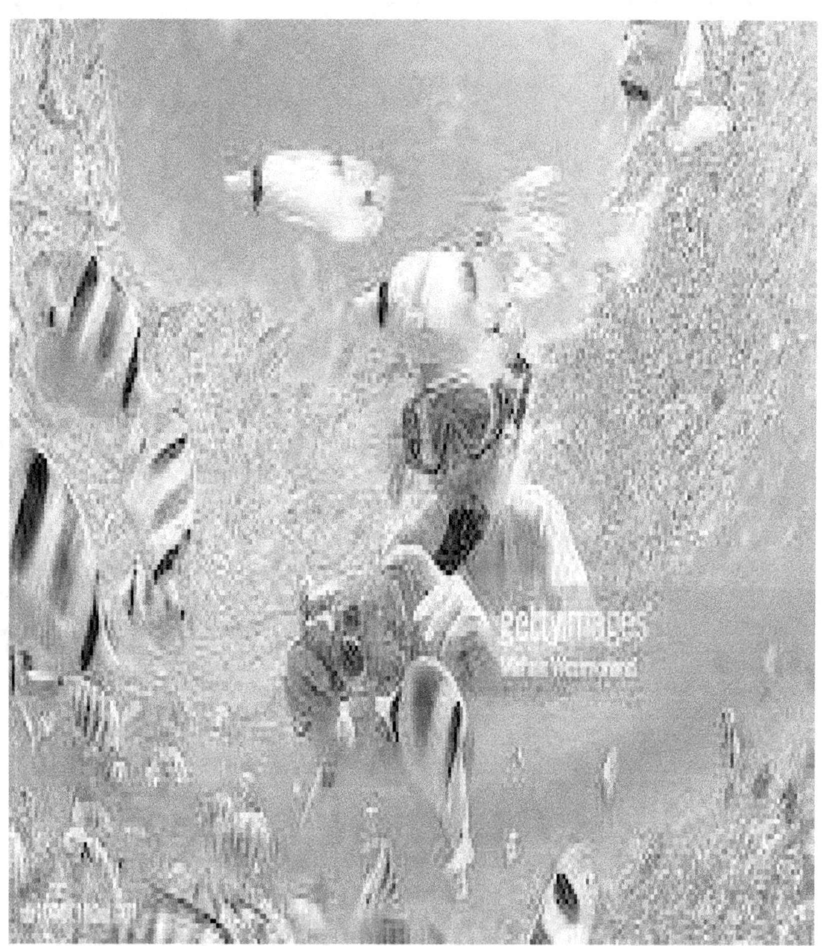

Snorkling in the Caribbean

came the feeling that this is a wonder of the world, missed as a young island native, but never the less I was able to enjoy it as an adult. So, as you can see, going to the beach was one of the best forms of relaxation both then and now. Sad to say, back then it was free, but now, this has all changed. For since it has become such a huge tourist spot, everyone must now pay to get into that beach as well as some of the other beaches. And this is an issue not taken lightly by the islanders. Now answer me this question. Who needs capitalizm taking over their fun virgin island lifestyle?

Another form of relaxation was not only visiting friends but also entertaining friends at home. Sometimes, I would take a stroll with them or sit up in or under a tree alone, eating a fruit or just doing nothing else but keeping cool. At other times though, just lying around the house because there was nothing better to do, but just to relax was all that I would do.

It is imperative to rest and relax. Life today has gotten to be so busy, that most people have to make such an effort to find the time to do this. But back in my youthful days it was second nature. No one thought of taking time off from work for relaxation. After school and work, even though there were other things incorporated into the day, people would in most cases, take time out for rest. This came naturally.

Another recreational activity was hiking. This was not a relaxation activity. It was more of an exercise activity good for both the body and the brain. It was done in groups and appreciated both for the socialization and overall good fun, chosen to be done for our own personal satisfaction. There were also other activities such as fishing, cricket, and football among others. Have you gotten the picture yet? Just a side note to say that ball games such as football are totally demonic. We should not be discussing them, watching them on any screen, applauding them or praising the winners. This game was formulated in hell, and to indulge yourself with it in any form shape or fashion, would cause you to be lost.

Relaxation and recreation promoted a stress-free environment; something we all need daily to encourage both good physical and psychological health. And it was most certainly a part of stress free island living.

PART THREE::: The Spritual

Embracing the Divine

And now it's time to talk about the focal point here. It pertains to my church life. It seemed as if almost everyone I knew was of a Christian persuasion. But occasionally I would meet people who believed otherwise. I saw only one lodge in the city which frankly gave me the creeps.

Whenever I heard gossip about people indulging in things pertaining to the dark side, it gave me a funny feeling in the pit of my stomach. I once had a family friend who paraded as a Christian, but she was just down right evil. She practiced witchcraft and influenced me to touch it as well. How sad. Let's just say that I have since confessed and repented, and the merciful Yahushua forgave and cleansed me from it. Thankfully I never have to deal with her ever again.

The Dominant Island Religion

Almost all families on this island were Catholic,

GJH 40

mine included. As a paganized Christian, I did my first holy communion, then confirmation, and attended all Catholic schools up until high school. My college experience was also at a Catholic University although I had already changed faith. At the age of thirteen, a family member tried to introduce me to a Bible based sabbath keeping religion. At first, I resisted but as I continued to argue, the Holy Spirit convicted me of that truth, so, I began to attend a village crusade, having to walk long distances by myself at night, with absolutely no fear of the dark. There were no streetlights along the road, but I was determined to attend those meetings with or without transportation. Based on what I was hearing at that crusade, I made a commitment to myself to continue attending to the end of those nightly meetings. There I became convinced that doctrinally it was the true religion since everything preached thus far was Biblically sound. So, I joined a baptismal class, got water baptized in a river, and gave the valedictorian speech for our class graduation. Needless to say, I left the Catholic church and lost some family support and some school authority support (the nuns). This was so because I rejected their religion.

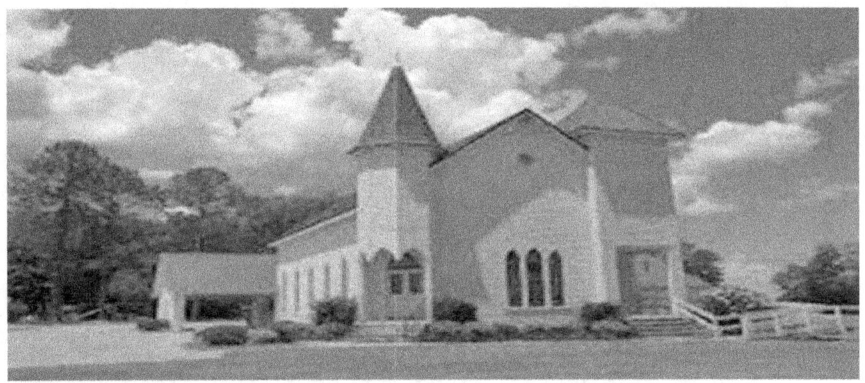

Sabbath Keeping Church

Much has happened to me since I joined that sabbath keeping church. But today I study my Bible independently, because instead of advancing in Biblical truth, as a church they have regressed. As a matter of fact, if any member is doing an in-depth study of the Bible, based on conference rules, that person must be disfellowshipped. However, I have made a conscious decision to move forward, gaining greater light as I study and worship at home with my family. My Bible studies have taken me deeper into greater truths, which I could never have imagined was in the Word. But I will continue to give credit to that small church, without which I could not have been where I am today spiritually. Praise the Most High!

PART FOUR::: An Open Initiative

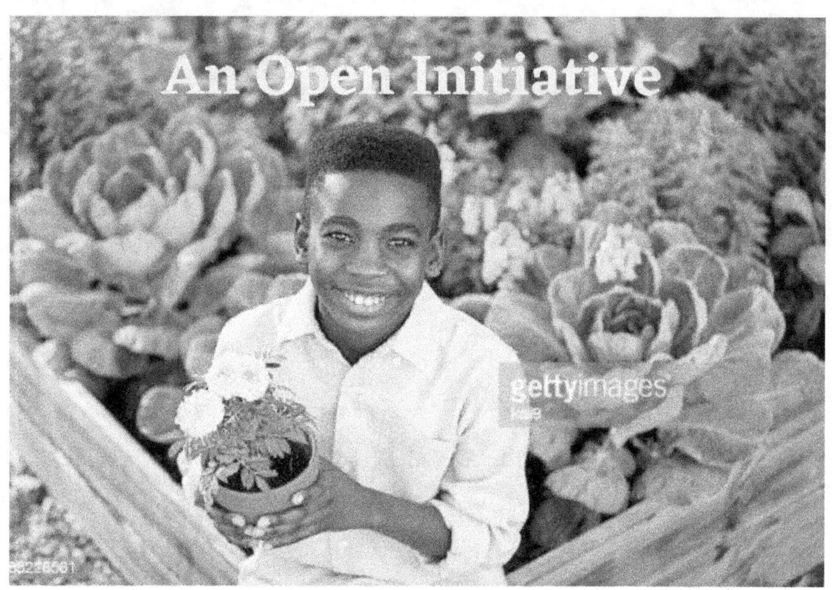

A Vegan Diet is Recommended to be Better Than a Flesh Diet.

And now it's time to pop the question. "Was there ever a time when while reading a book- any book, where someone gave you an open invitation, to take what is in front of you and live it out in your daily life?" Well, if you haven't had this happen to you yet, today is the day that you are being given such an invitation. I call this invite, "An Open Initiative" to take control of your health. To take the bull by the horn and win the fight to either keep or transform yourself with a glow, that whenever others see you, they may stop and ask you to give them your secret for looking the way you do. **Health is Wealth!** And now I give you what I call **"An Open Initiative."**

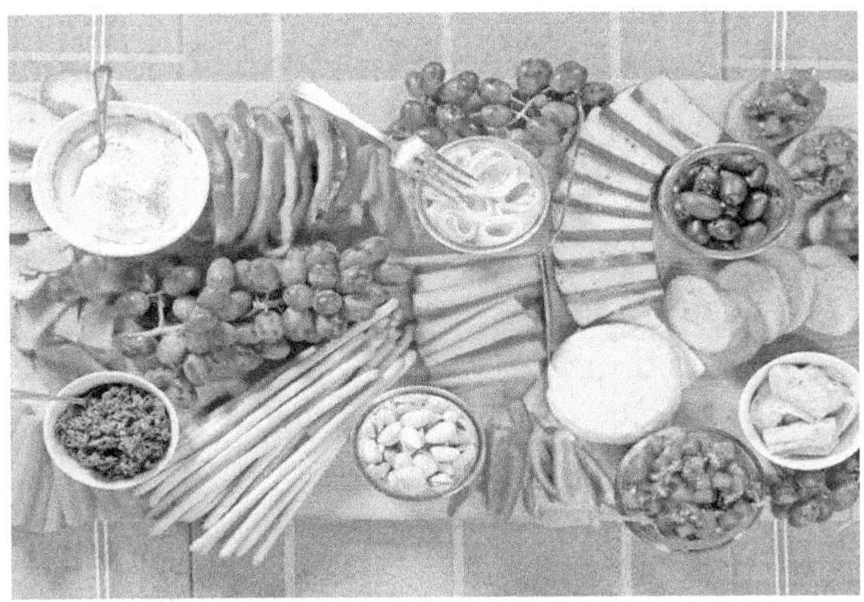

Vegan Grazing Table

Three Distinct Causes of Diseases

Disease has been identified in three different categories -- hereditary, communicative, and self-acquired. Since this is so, then there must be three kinds of sin based on the transgression of three laws which are i- Sin against The Most High, ii- sin against our fellowman, and iii – sin against our own selves. These laws are written, not only in the Decalogue in Exodus 20:3-17 KJV, but also in the Mosaic Law, both found in the Old Testament.

Since this is so then sinning against God, which is the first type mentioned, causes a hereditary curse, the kind that passes down unto the third and fourth generation of them that hate Him, Exodus. 20:5 KJV.

The second type mentioned, which is sinning against others, brings communicative diseases or an unfortunate consequence. Such was the case of King Uzziah. He attempted to burn incense in the Temple which was something that only the priests were allowed to do. When they tried to prevent him from doing this, he became angry and was immediately struck with leprosy, 2 Chronicles 26:20-23 KJV. Another example was in the case of Daniel. This case in point is more of a judgment than a disease, nevertheless, it is the sort of thing that happens when we do things to others spitefully. At some point, it brings with it a judgement where, instead of the person we are trying to hurt falling, we can end up falling into our own pit. In this instance, the princes and presidents of King Darius of Media and Persia, sort to find fault against Daniel out of jealousy; so they "assembled together to the king, and said thus unto him, King Darius, live for ever. All the presidents of the kingdom, the governors, and the princes, the counsellors, and the captains, have consulted together to establish a royal statute, and to make a firm decree, that whosoever shall ask a petition *of any God or man for thirty days,* save of thee, O king, he shall be cast into the den of lions. Now, O king, establish the decree, and sign the writing, that it be not changed, according to the law of the Medes and Persians, which altereth not. Wherefore king Darius signed the writing and the decree," Daniel 6:6-9 KJV. These men did this out of jealousy because the king, who trusted Daniel had put him in a very high position in the kingdom. But when their plan was executed not only did it fail, but once Daniel was taken out of the den, they were cast in and immediately devoured by those hungry lions. It is a very unwise thing to sin against others or against their children.

The third type of disease or discomfort mentioned here happens when a person sins against himself, like in the case of sexual immorality. The Apostle Paul advises us to "Flee fornication." Every sin that a man doeth is without the body; but he that committeth fornication sinneth against his own body," 1 Corinthians 6:18 KJV. We also offend our bodies by breaking the eight laws of health, particularly with regards to eating unclean foods or taking various forms of drugs; particularly illegal drugs. Our bodies are the temple of the Holy Spirit. When we sin against our own body, we reap what we sow!

If a person is suffering from a hereditary disease, he will, without the help of the Most High, be unable to do anything about it. Only by strict obedience to Biblical commandments and laws can a cure be realized, along with belief in the promise given in the third commandment which reads, "And shewing mercy unto thousands of them that love me, and keep my commandments," Exodus 20:6 KJV.

Regarding the person suffering from a communicative disease, in order to affect a cure, he must forgive and repent of the sin, and begin walking in the counsel of Yahushua HaMashiach which says, "All things whatsoever ye that men should do to you, do ye even so to them," Matthew, 7:12 KJV.

Lastly, one of the most difficult sins to conquer is the sin against self. Although it might appear to be the easiest to control, this one can in most cases be the most difficult to overcome. Here is where self-control is needed, notwithstanding the fact that with every evil act committed, there is a   demon attached to it. Some demons can be stubborn unwanted guest, "howbeit this kind goeth not out but by prayer and fasting," Mathew 17:21 KJV.

Choose Life

For those who might not know what's causing their discomfort, it can be because that person is not living a more simplified life. Maybe he is committing a variety of sins or just eating too many unhealthy foods or even taking too many unhealthy things into the body at the same time. For instance, a drug user might be taking both prescribe as well as illegal drugs in combination with each other. Here is where living a more simplified life becomes most important. Just

knowing the cause of a particular disease, and what can be done to bring about a cure, will be the determining factor as to whether the person wins the battle to preserve health and life.
There is no wisdom in looking at what you might consider a minor ailment to be less serious than a bigger problem. Let me give you an example. Sometime in the past, when I first moved into a high-rise condominium, I would experience headaches every day. What I found strange is that my daughter complained of the same discomfort. I questioned what was causing it, because it seemed as if I was doing everything correctly regarding taking care of myself, and so was she. I had not too long moved into the building, and since I was on the seventh floor, I didn't think much about not opening all the windows.

One day, as I began to open those windows, I noticed that the headaches were beginning to subside. That is when I knew that the reason for my headaches was simply because there was not enough oxygen coming into the house. It was just that one thing causing such discomfort. The health law which I broke was that of having a lack of oxygen. And because my life was simple, I was able to easily identify the problem and fix it. This is just one example of not cluttering what you do, so that if something goes wrong, the problem can easily be identified and attended to.

The Human Body is a Machine

Some people, especially men have a tendency to take care of their vehicles with more love than they take care of their own bodies. Some men clean it every day, and wash it once a week, maybe twice depending on the weather. They keep the gas tank with sufficient gas so that they don't stall while driving. They check the brake fluid, the engine oil, and the radiator, and without hesitation they pull over to see what's happening if the check engine light should come on. If our cars are so important to us, our bodies should be considered even more important and should be treated with way more respect.

The human body is the most complicated machine. Therefore, we should eat only the healthiest foods to keep from starving and drink enough water to keep from becoming dehydrated. If we are depleted of energy, we can stop functioning and die. Unlike the car, we cannot go to the auto repair shop to get ourselves up and running again. Once the heart stops beating, the body dies. You can service any broken-down old machine to get it working again, but you cannot do that with the human body once it dies. If you want to live a long and healthy life, whereby your cells can rejuvenate themselves, then you must take care of your blood, because "the life of the flesh is in the blood," Leviticus 17:11 KJV. If you want good blood, then you must eat good food. And for meat eaters, be wise and study the book of Leviticus chapter 11 KJV, which tells exactly what should and should not be eaten. A good diet, along with keeping the other eight laws of health, which will be discussed a little later, is what builds the blood and keeps the body functioning well. The blood not only provides nutrients to, but it also removes waist from the body. "The days of our years are three score years and ten (seventy years)," Psalms 90:10 KJV. There is an old saying that "an ounce of prevention is better than a whole pound of cure."

Therefore, why wait until something goes wrong to address your health? Begin to treat your body better than you treat your car. Don't depend on surgery to do for you what the auto shop will do to replace broken car parts, for then it might be too late to continue living. Our bodies are beautifully made, and if we do our part to maintain it, the Most High will do His portion and bless us with even more years than He has originally promised.

Nature is Our Instructor

Nature teaches us how to take care of our bodies. Take for instance plants; they never do well in soil depleted of nutrients, nor do they thrive in climates not favorable to them. A tropical plant will not grow in cold climates with fridged temperatures. As we look at the portion of nature pertaining to plants and animals, we notice that plants can make their own food from inorganic raw materials, while animals, not being able to synthesize their own food, must rely on other sources, particularly plant and animal matter. The emphasis here is to encourage the reader to ingest only organic plant material. A flesh diet is a secondhand diet: therefore, it is much better to provide the body with the nutrients it needs firsthand, thus bypassing the meat diet in exchange for an organic vegan diet. A faulty meat diet can be a catalyst for cancer and other diseases. If the animal is sick and you cook it and bring it to the dinner table, this will cause you to also be sick. At one point in time, if you told the average person that they did not need to eat meat to maintain health, and that it was not the best diet for anyone, they would have practically laughed you to scorn. But in recent years, many, including athletes, have transitioned to eating at least a vegetarian diet and in some cases a vegan diet. This is so because of the sicknesses that have been known to be derived from eating a flesh diet. Learn to cook these meals for yourself, it will benefit you.

When I first made the transition from eating a flesh diet to a vegetarian diet, I didn't fully understand how to do it. But I was willing to learn. I didn't tell myself that this was too difficult for me to do. I persisted without full knowledge. Until one day, the Holy Spirit impressed upon me to cook everything else that I usually cook, except for meat. That is when the light bulb went on in my head, and I began to do just that. Once I did this, I noticed that I felt lighter, and what made it even better was that my children never missed meat. They were contented, and as a family, we were eventually able to transition from a vegetarian diet to eating a well-balanced nutritious vegan diet. If I can do it, you can too. So be willing and go for it. This can be accomplished!

Eating poorly can result in various health complications, but if we take care of ourselves from the inside, it will be reflected on the outside. We will have less malaise, and our faces will glow with unsurpassed youth regardless of our age. Make-up is never the answer to not looking good. It might cover a few things presently, but eventually as we continue using it, the glow will fade, thus causing more harm than good. Another area for consideration is how we are to keep our surroundings. It is important to keep both our bodies and living areas clean.

"Cleanliness is indeed next to godliness." ----John Wesley.

Uncleanness is a catalyst for diseases. First take

away the cause of the problem and that will automatically eliminate the problem.

Let Food be Your Medicine

In most cases, except if the person has gotten into an accident, the cause of a particular health problem might just be attributed to what we ingest. If you eat or drink the wrong things, it can result in a wrong circumstance. Take for instance drinking alcohol. I knew quite a few people from the islands who ended their own lives by drinking alcohol (rum). Others have gotten diabetic by eating too many sweets and desserts. Some people suffer from having an upset stomach because of eating the wrong food combinations, while many treat water as if it is an enemy and end up constipated and dehydrated, from not drinking enough of it daily. I used to not drink enough water, but I have since corrected that. And I continue to try not to eat incorrectly combined foods anymore.

Commercially prepared foods and fast foods are also something that I will never recommend for eating, since we don't know exactly how they are being prepared, and what ingredients are included in making them. These are deceitful foods, and eating them along with drinking insufficient water daily are two of the main causes of constipation. The first thing I would do to solve this problem would be to change my eating habits and increase my daily fluid intake. While growing up, parents gave children such harsh purges, where you stayed using the bathroom all day. Some people nowadays even do colon cleansing; something I don't recommend. I always tell people that when Yahushua was on earth, nowhere in the account says that He took a purge or did a colon cleanse, and He was never ill. That is because He ate a balanced diet. He did not overeat, and He drank enough water. Not discounting the fact that according to the Book of Genesis, Methuselah lived to the good old age of nine hundred sixty-nine years old (969), while others, though their lives were shorter, exceeded our present-day lifespan by many years. We were not created to be sick, but we must do our part to maintain our health, and we can!

In order to supply the body with the proper materials for building and maintenance, we cannot eat junk food. Those who do this cause their body to become deficient and not able to function well. This has long-lasting effects, which, although not felt immediately, will definitely be felt eventually. The problem with this though is that by the time these effects are felt, it might be too late to reverse any negatives derived from unhealthy eating habits. An onset of illness is a notice from the body to warn us to wake up and amend our daily living habits. Why wait until you get so sick that you end up with an emergency at the doctor's office or undergoing an operation at the hospital? It is better never to compromise your health. The most important asset you own is your health. For as the saying goes,

"Health is Wealth." ----American philosopher Ralph Waldo Emerson.

Sometimes it is necessary for medication to be administered, although I believe that every disease can be treated and cured with herbal remedies, instead of synthetics drugs. The most important aspect of healing is to always keep in mind that any illness in nature can be treated by nature. Some examples can be just a common cold ranging all the way to a more serious lung complication. Lung problems can be treated with herbs, but the case must be dealt with at the early onset.
Another case is that of hypo and hyperthyroidism.

With these illnesses, once blood work is done, and you know exactly what needs to be treated based on the lab results, a strict regimen using the correct herbs can be administered daily to eliminate the problem with success.

Yet another problem is body pain. Something causes pain. It may be caused by a structural problem in the body which can be more difficult to treat, and you might need to visit a Chiro practitioner, or it can be caused by constipation which is way easier to treat.
Still yet, one of the most common pains is a headache, which might just mean that you need more oxygen in your space. So, if you would just open the windows and let some fresh air in, then you will be fine. But what do most people do? They run to the doctor who will only prescribe synthetic medication. Hence the problem gets worse, while the doctor gets rich.

But, there are some instances where medication is needed. Take for example if a person gets into a sudden accident and needs stitches to rejoin the flesh, then yes. Another case is this. If a woman is in labor, she might need an epidural or a local anesthesia to help deliver the baby. Nevertheless, overall, health issues can be successfully addressed, by using a well-tailored diet to counteract that ailment, or the problem can be treated with herbal remedies.

Never overlook the fact that the human body is made up of minerals found in food. Therefore, by eating correctly, nature is able to maintain the body in a perfect condition, but we must always, and in all instances, co-operate with nature.

Eating a Flesh Diet

In the beginning God said to the man: "Behold I have given you every herb bearing seed which is upon the face of all the earth, and every tree, in the which is the fruit of a tree yielding seed; to you it shall be for meat." Genesis 1:29 KJV.

Initially, there were no meat eaters in the Garden of Eden or even after, when the pair were put out of the Garden. Even though they now dealt with thorns and thistles which made life less easy to bear, Adam was instructed to till the ground for by the sweat of his brow he was to eat bread, Genesis 3:18 KJV.

It was after Yahuveh destroyed the world by flood waters, that He gave Noah and his family permission to eat flesh food. He allowed them to eat only clean meats; details of which are found written in book of Leviticus chapter 11 KJV. Then the average length of life immediately dropped significantly to somewhere between one to two hundred years. Most likely, the Most High wanted to shorten human life by allowing us to eat meat. People before the flood lived over 900 years since they were vegetarians, but after the flood and the introduction of a meat diet, the age of men dropped drastically to around a little over hundred years. Yahuveh intended to restrict the life span of evil doers to limit their wickedness. Thus, the short life would serve only as a time of testing, enough for men to make eternal decisions either for Heaven, or against the Most High for Hell. These were the instructions, "Every moving thing that liveth shall be meat for you; even as the green herb have I given you all things. But flesh with the life thereof, which is the blood thereof, shall ye not eat. And surely your blood of your lives will I require; at the <u>hand</u> of every **beast** will I require it, and at the <u>hand</u> of **man**; at the <u>hand</u> of every **man's brother** will I require the life of man, Genesis 9:3-5 KJV.

The dietary requirement for holy living is a plan-based diet, which can be proven from the Bible itself.

Speaking of John the Baptist, it was said of Him

that "he shall be great in the sight of the Lord, and shall drink neither wine nor strong drink; and he shall be filled with the Holy Ghost, even from his mother's womb. Luke 1:15 KJV. Hence, his was a strict vegetarian diet, "……his meat
was locusts and wild honey," Mathew 3:4 KJV. About the children of Israel after they left Egypt to go into the promise land, they "did eat manna forty years, until they came to a land inhabited; they did eat manna, until they came unto the borders of the land of Canaan," Exodus 16:35 KJV.

And now let us take a look at the account of Daniel and his friends once taken into Babylonian captivity while they were in the house of King Nebuchadnezzar which reads, " But Daniel purposed in his heart that he would not defile himself with the portion of the king's meat, nor with the wine which he drank: therefore he requested of the prince of the eunuchs that he might not defile himself. Now God had brought Daniel into favour and tender love with the prince of the eunuchs. And the prince of the eunuchs said unto Daniel, I fear my lord the   king, who hath appointed your meat and your drink for why should he see your faces worse liking than the children which are of your sort? then shall ye make me endanger my head to the king. Then said Daniel to Melzar, whom the prince of the eunuchs had set over Daniel, Hananiah, Mishael, and Azariah, Prove thy servants, I beseech thee, ten days; and let them give us pulse to eat, and water to drink. Then let our countenances be looked upon before thee, and the countenance of the children that eat of the portion of the king's meat: and as thou seest, deal with thy servants. So he consented to them in this matter, and proved them ten days. And at the end of ten days their countenances appeared fairer and fatter in flesh than all the children which did eat the portion of the king's meat. Thus Melzar took away the portion of their meat, and the wine that they should drink; and gave them pulse. As for these four children, God gave them knowledge and skill in all learning and wisdom: and Daniel had understanding in all visions and dreams. Now at the end of the days that the king had said he should bring them in, then the prince of the eunuchs brought them in before Nebuchadnezzar. And the king communed with them; and among them all was found none like Daniel, Hananiah, Mishael, and Azariah: therefore stood they before the king. And in all matters of wisdom and understanding, that the king enquired of them, he found them ten times better than all the magicians and astrologers that were in all his realm," Daniel 1: 8-20 KJV. Vegetarianism is a holy dietary requirement, and in the case of Daniel who showed himself faithful to The Most High, he became fatter of flesh, meaning healthier, more so than everyone else who ate at the king's table.

Vegetarianism

The vegetarian can supply all his dietary needs, living comfortably and healthily on vegetables, beans, fruits, nuts, and grains. Not all these items need to be cooked, and whatever can be eaten raw should be eaten raw. It is, however, necessary to cook some of these, as they cannot be otherwise digested. When making the switch from a meat diet to a vegetarian or vegan diet, it is better to eat what you can raw. Not all vegetables can and should be eaten raw, but those that can be steamed should not be cooked. The nutritional value of steamed food is greater than that of cooked food. Don't force yourself to eat everything raw; that will not be wise, but as much as possible eat uncooked vegetables, since they hold a greater nutritional value than cooked veggies. Chew well. Remember that digestion begins in the mouth. I know that it is customary to cook your food, but as a vegetarian or vegan, to get the best out of everything you eat, and to preserve a healthy-looking demeanor, you must begin to make this change gradually. Eat raw and cooked food together to prevent the lining of the stomach from becoming irritated. Use seasonings in moderation. There is no need to eliminate salt from your diet. You need it to maintain a fluid balance. Seasoned food is enjoyed much more than eating bland food, and if you are not accustomed to eating raw food, then begin with small amounts, just as long as you begin.

Many items such as beans, nuts, grains and fruits can be dried for out of season use and export. And certain fruits which do not grow in a particular climate can also be exported to be enjoyed in other countries too. For instance, when I lived in the Caribbean, I looked forward to the months when apples were imported from foreign countries, because for some reason, we were unable to grow our own in that warm climate. The concern with vegetarianism, however, is that when meat eaters make the switch to a plant-based diet, they fail to look healthy, thus giving vegetarianism a bad name. The problem here is not with the food, it is with the fact that these people don't bother taking the time to learn how to prepare their meals. A good suggestion would be to purchase a cookbook in this area and begin to practice how to prepare meals without meat. Practice makes perfect, and pretty soon you will realize that you not only don't even miss your previous diet, but that you will never want to return to it, because you have now found a pearl of great price; a better diet without the worry of becoming sick. Anything can follow you from the supermarket to your dinner table. You never know what's in meat, exactly what type of fresh it is and where it came from. You don't know if it is genetically modified, if it was produced in a lab thus making it artificial meat or if it is cancerous. So don't take chances. Change your diet and save your life.

The types of foods and their groups needed for a balanced diet are grouped below. If they are proportioned correctly, there should be no problem in maintaining a well-balanced diet.

Approximately 80% of your diet should be of the first eight classes of food. (Group 1). 20% of your diet should be of the second three classes of foods (Group 2). And the rest of your diet should be of the third class, consisting of seasonings (Group 3).

<u>Group one: 80% of the Diet</u>

This portion must consist of the foods in this group:

1st -- Leaves (watercress, beet tops, spinach lettuce, parsley, cabbage, broccoli, cauliflower, chard.)
2nd -- Stalks (Celery, rhubarb, asparagus.)
3rd -- Herbal Fruits (pineapple, okra, eggplant, peppers, string beans, tomatoes.)
4th -- Tubers (carrots, potatoes, radishes, onions, yams, beets, turnips.)
5th -- Cucurbits (squash, melons, cucumbers, pumpkins.)
6th -- Tree Fruits (peaches, dates, bananas oranges, pomegranates, olives, avocados.)
7th -- Vine Fruits (berries, grapes.)
8th -- Dairy Products (for vegetarians).

Entering Wedge Society of America et al. 29 – 30.
GJH 66

Group Two: 20% of the Diet

Only about 20% of one's diet should be made up of the foods in this group:

1st -- Grains (oats, rice, corn, rye, wheat, barley, etc.)
2nd -- Legumes (beans, lentils, peas, etc.)
3rd -- Nuts (pecans, coconuts, almonds, walnuts, chestnuts, etc.)

Group Three: Seasonings for all Foods

All foods may be seasoned with the foods of this group:

1st -- Oils (olive oil, soybean oil, sesame oil, nut oils, cottonseed oil.)
2nd -- Sweets (honey, raw sugar, maple sugar, sorghum.)
3rd – Herbs (parsley, chives, basil, coriander, cardamon, celery, oregano, thyme, pepper, paprika, bay-leaf, fenugreek, ginger, oregano and any other of your liking.)

Entering Wedge Society of America et al. 29 - 30.

Combining Foods

As someone who cooks regularly, food combination is something that I find myself doing without even giving it a second thought. Needless to say, not all food combinations are good for the stomach. One such combination is <u>fruits mixed with vegetables</u>. But the emphasis here is not so much on what is bad for us to do, but more so on what is good. In most cases, fruits should not be mixed with vegetables, but in some cases, they can be mixed at mealtime. For instance. most people consider tomato a vegetable, but it is a fruit, another fruit is lemon and yet another is avocado. These are just some examples of fruits mixed into our salad daily with no negative effect.

Some fruits, however, should never be mixed with vegetables since vegetables break down way faster once they reach the stomach. For instance, oranges should not be mixed with carrots while strawberries can be mixed with spinach in salads and smoothies.

Other food combinations besides only fruits and vegetables that offer unbelievable health benefits are:-

Tomatoes and olive oil

Rice and beans

Leafy green vegetables and lemon juice

Oatmeal and blueberries

Cereals and berries

Garlic and onions

Crushed walnuts over broccoli

Vegetables have many fat-soluble vitamins, like A, D, E, and K which means that it is okay to sauté them in **organic extra virgin olive oil** since they need fat to be absorbed,"

<u>Fruit and fruit combination</u>: - Not all fruits must be eaten together, for instance, banana which can act as a laxative should not be combined with guava which can cause constipation. I can personally tell you about guava. In the West Indies, our land was loaded with all different species of them. Lemon, which is acidic, should not be mixed with sweet papaya. And melons should only be eaten with melons as they are digested more rapidly than other fruits. These fruits are very refreshing to eat, but for the best

benefits, eat only those that are compatible together. This will avoid gas bloating and acid reflux.

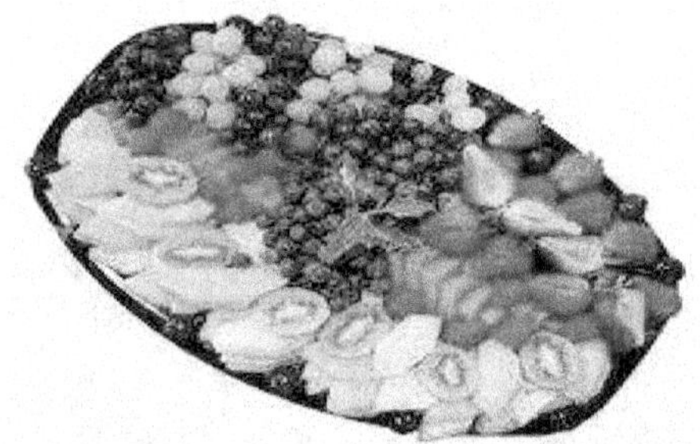

<u>Protein and carbohydrate combination</u>: - These are two different types of digestion: an acid digestion for proteins (beans and veggie cheese) and an alkaline digestion for carbohydrates (sugars and starches). Now let's look at it from a practical plant base perspective. As for me, I find it virtually impossible not to combine **proteins** and **carbohydrates** in the same meal. Most foods contain some **protein**, some **carbohydrates,** and some fats. For instance, if I cook a macaroni pie, the ingredients contained of course are pasta, but I must also include milk and butter with various seasonings, plus a little oil in the container to bake it in. This was a staple and delicacy at every Sunday family meal when I was living in the Caribbean, and no one ever complained of discomfort after lunch. I also make it now for my family using all the same

ingredients. The only difference is that everything is plant based. All things considered, I would have to just leave this one up to the individual's discretion, and my only advice would be to do everything in moderation.

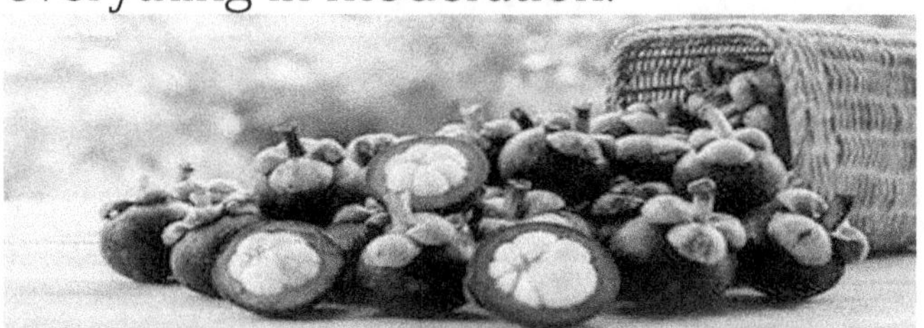

<u>Combining home grown foods with imported foods</u>: - There is absolutely no problem eating imported foods as long as they are kept clean and safe. Most likely, they will lose some of their nutrients during travel from one country to the next, but the advantage here is the variety brought to the table by foods that cannot be produced locally at home. For example, even though I now live in a cold climate, I still like eating all those West Indian foods. Why can't I still have my dasheen, cassava and tania. There is nothing unhealthy about sharing the taste of the islands with people of a colder climate.

Locally grown food is full of flavor since the crops are picked at their peak of ripeness. They keep 100% of their nutrients as they are harvested and eaten seasonally. So go ahead and add imported foods to locally grown foods on your menus. This will provide not only variety, but many health benefits, as you enjoy your favorite meals with both friends and family.

Summer foods and winter foods are very different. Plants grow in the summer and lay dormant in the winter. In the summer, various varieties of fresh fruits and vegetables are available at relatively good prices, but in the winter, it is difficult to find a huge variety of these foods. When the weather is hot, we often begin craving lighter, colder food and drinks to keep cool. But in the winter, we tend to eat warm foods, with cravings for hot soups higher in calories to help keep us warm. There are a few reasons why nutritional needs change from season to season, and much of it is centered around the weather. Because there is less sunlight in the winter months, it would be wise to eat foods that are a good source of Vitamin D, needed to help the body absorb and retain calcium and phosphorus; both critical for maintaining and building healthy bones. Flaxseeds, chia seeds, and walnuts are good sources of Omega -3 fatty acids to help the skin look less dry. And vitamin C, derived from

Cruciferous vegetables (broccoli, brussels sprouts cabbage, cauliflower), tomatoes, citrus and white potatoes; help boost the immune system to fight off colds during the winter months.

While freshly picked fruits and vegetables are available in the summer, dried foods, for example beans, canned and preserved foods are also available in the winter. Canned foods are not the healthiest though. Our diet doesn't change too much from season to season, but we do eat a little heavier in the winter to stay warm. Fruit is a summer food, designed to keep the body cool. The person who lives in a warm climate is able to eat more fresh foods, but a person who lives in a cold climate needs to eat more of the dry, preserved, concentrated, heat-producing foods with greater caloric benefits. These different kinds of foods are all necessary, however, some are more specific to a particular country.
My all-time favorite foods are summer foods consisting of fruits and vegetables, and particularly my favorite fruit: The Julie Mango!

Health Reform

Health Reform is a process of change involving the who, what and how of a person's lifestyle. Health reform implies not only fundamental changes, but purposeful changes as well. When I say fundamental, I mean that the basic everyday things a person do, must change. And when I say purposeful, I mean that the person must be single minded and determined, not second guessing himself. These changes do not have to be difficult if you begin to make them, by taking baby steps. After all, everyone must creep before they walk, don't they? And this is how I unintentionally mapped out my own reform. First it was in the area of food, then in the area of dressing and finally in the area of my overall demeanor, all of which took practice on a daily basis. Let no one fool you. No one can change their way overnight. Change takes time. When I began to reform, I decided on the holistic approach, meaning not only in food, but also in my wardrobe along with my Biblical beliefs. I did not know everything. Most things I had to learn, and that took time. Of myself, I had no rules to follow, so what I did was to follow Biblical rules. Where food was concerned, it was with the Edenic diet when I

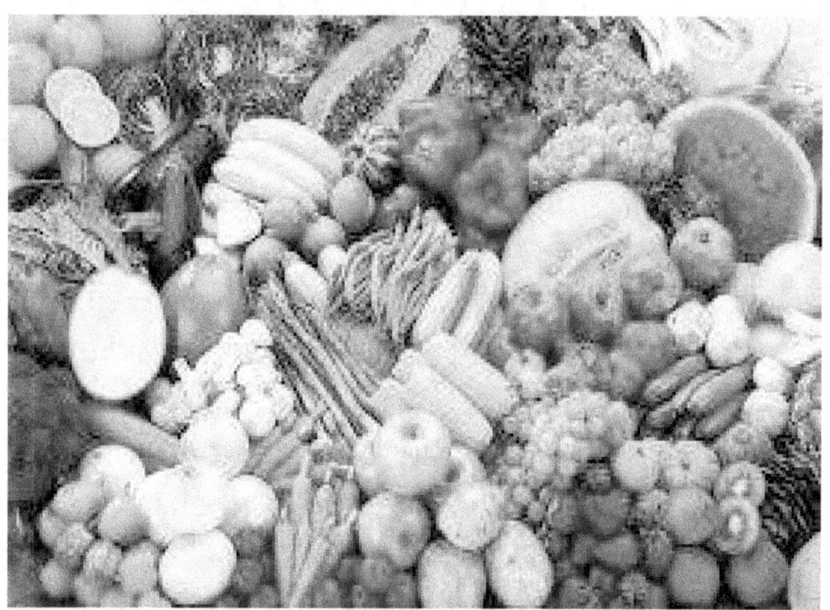

Fruits, Nuts, Grains and Vegetables

began to exclude eating meat. And where clothing was concerned, it was by the instructions given in the statute law of Moses, for example "Thou shalt **not** wear a garment of divers sorts, as of **woolen** and **linen** together," Deuteronomy 22:11 KJV. Hence, now I wear mostly100% linen clothing, a much-appreciated change. This fabric makes my skin feel so much cooler. These though are not the only changes I made. I still continue to make changes by learning directly from the Most High and from His prophets, but not everyone is the same. People learn in various ways. However, the area of reform that proved the most difficult for me was in that of separation.

Isolation can mean different things to different people. In my case it was for separation and the set-apart life. Health does not only mean physical health. It also means spiritual and mental health as well. Don't get me wrong. This does not mean that I now live like a hermit, oh no. I actually live in a house with nine other family members, but this separation took me away from the city and into the country, based on religious instruction, given by our present-day prophetess. Once I did this with my family, I found that living a reformed life got way easier. I no longer had to worry about the day-to-day distractions experienced in the city, which feels so good, so much so that many times when I pray, even though transition to country living is still somewhat a bit difficult, I thank Yahuveh and His Son Yahushua, for putting me where I can breathe so much fresh air in quietness. I thank them for putting me among the trees.

The Word and Nature are Divine Light

The psalmist David says in Psalms 19:1-4 KJV that "The heavens declare the glory of God; and the firmament sheweth his handywork. Day unto day uttereth speech, and night unto night sheweth knowledge. There is no speech nor language, where their voice is not heard. Their line is gone out through all the earth, and their words to the end of the world. In them hath he set a tabernacle for the sun."

In only these first four verses, David was able to, without doubt, show that both The WORD and NATURE are our divine teachers. There is no need to move outside of them to learn the necessary things in life. Some other Biblical verses to consider in this context are: - "Verily, verily, I say unto you, Except a corn of wheat fall into the ground and die, it abideth alone: but if it die, it bringeth forth much fruit," John 12:24 KJV. Genesis 8:22 KJV reads, "While the earth remaineth, seedtime and harvest, and cold and heat, and summer and winter, and day and night shall not cease." Job 12: 7-9 KJV says, "But ask now the beasts, and they shall teach thee; and the fowls of the air, and they shall tell thee: Or speak to the earth, and it shall teach thee: and the fishes of the sea shall declare unto thee. Who knoweth not in all these that the hand of the LORD hath wrought this?" And Yahushua, while on earth referred to His own creative work when He said, "And why take ye thought for raiment? Consider the lilies of the field, how they grow; they toil not, neither do they spin: And yet I say unto you, That even Solomon in all his glory was not arrayed like one of these," Mathew 6:28, 29 KJV.

Now, since Romans 1:20 KJV says, "his invisible attributes, namely, his eternal power and divine nature, have been clearly perceived, ever since the creation of the world, in the things that have been made." Then the wisdom here is to understand that the same Person who created everything in nature by His Word, has also created exactly what we should eat in nature by His Word. See Genesis 1:29,30 KJV. and Leviticus 11 KJV.

His Word provides. Therefore, these instructions are valid. THE WORD and NATURE speak with authority. And if we decide that we will turn away from them and do our own thing, then we have with eyes wide open, willingly walked away from The Creator and nature, hence doing own selves a great dis-service, by living independently of the authority of Divine Light. Let us therefore heed our instructors so "that thou mayest prosper and be in health, even as thy soul prospereth," 3 John 1:2 KJV.

Wisdom and the Appetite

Overeating can be looked upon as just being plain greedy. There is absolutely no reason to consume more calories than are needed to produce the energy to carry out daily physical activities. This is a common problem, existing especially among sedentary folks. Obesity is not pretty. If we eat only what we need, chances are that gastrointestinal problems will be avoided. Since the average stomach holds about a liter (a quart), it is a good idea not to stretch the stomach by eating more than it is supposed to hold. The stomach is about the size of a fist, but not because it can expand means that we always have to follow our cravings. It is not wise to go looking for health problems.

Overeating is one of the areas in which I am usually forced to practice self-control. I must say though, that lately I have been doing quite well, since for spiritual reasons, blocks of time have been given to fasting. This helps, but there have been instances, even in childhood where binge eating caused me so many health issues. These included vomiting and indigestion, heartburn, acid reflux, nausea, gas, and bloating. There were also instances where my stomach felt overloaded resulting in a feeling of laziness.

To grow and build muscles, one needs to eat enough of the right foods but not overeat. And as people get older, having a slower metabolism; energy levels are also reduced. Thus, food intake must also be reduced. The greater reduction of food though, is most apparent in those having a more sedentary lifestyle and as we begin to age.

Not because the refrigerator is full, it means that we must eat it all in one day. Everyone cannot eat. Some sick people must be tube fed. But those who are healthy and still have this privilege, should "……eat to the satisfying of his soul…....:" Proverbs 13:25 KJV, and thank the Most High for the preserving of health which still affords them to do so. Eat to live and not the other way around. A good practice like I always say, is to eat breakfast as a king, lunch as a prince and dinner as a pauper. A narrower slogan still would simply be to eat breakfast like a king, skip lunch and eat dinner like a pauper. Many of us have been taught to eat three meals a day, but eating two meals a day would not only keep the body feeling lighter, but bring an added benefit of keeping ourselves healthier. And our stomachs will thank us for it. All in all, the Good Book sums it up quite nicely which is to "…… eat in due season, for strength, and not for drunkenness!" Ecclesiastes 10:17 KJV.

Some people like to nibble. If their mouth is not chewing on something they don't feel good. I guess chewing gum was invented to accommodate those kinds of people but know this; nibbling will eventually injure you.

Most people like to snack on something sweet. Sugar however, if it is not brushed off the teeth soon enough after snacking, this can result in cavities and bleeding gums, as your gums begin to recede. Here's the deal: carbohydrates in your snacks are converted to acids by bacteria that live in your mouth. Even though your mouth is home to these bacteria, they can still begin to break down the minerals out of your teeth, and cause cavities.

If you snack around the clock, then your mouth is never clean, as the average person would not even think of washing harmful acids and food particles out of the mouth, after eating their favorite snack.

Some sweets that tend to stick to the teeth, for

example toffees, candies, cookies, chips, and sticky fruit bars are not good snacks. These, although they might give you a quick energy boost, are   filled with processed sugar offering no nutritional value. So, where I am concerned, they are nice to run away from. And beverages such as caffeinated coffee and tea, sodas, and those dreaded energy drinks and snacks are just as guilty, causing the same, if not worse health problems. I find that children have a bad habit of snacking. I was once a child too and had good fun with lots of candies, bubble gum, tamarind ball, caser balls, toffies, and the list goes on. The problem here was that no one bothered to check up on my dental health, so I began getting cavities and losing my teeth at a very early age. By enjoying all these sweets, I placed myself at risk for poor dental health and bad breath at a very early stage in life.

Many people snack because they are bored, thus quickly adding up calories, resulting in weight gain and risking their health. Just picture yourself eating and leaving a little food on your plate, then adding a little more a few hours after that, and so on and so on. Never really finishing eating that plate completely and then not washing that plate, but adding more food to it the following day, then eating that food, and repeating same the process all over again. Naturally, your food would begin to break down even from the plate with a bad smell. In like manner, when you snack continuously, you cause fermentation in your stomach, and this results in, guess what? It causes both an acidic smell and foul-smelling gas. In other words, you literally make bad air.

To avoid this, you must stop snacking and give your stomach a chance to do the work that it was designed to do properly. By not emptying from meal to meal, the stomach ferments with a buildup of toxins. If you feel hungry between meals, do what I do. Practice drinking water. This will both hydrate and flush you until you feel light and comfortable on the inside.

Another dangerous habit, one that I have been guilty of, is that of eating just before bedtime. As a result, digestion continues while asleep resulting in unpleasant dreams, even nightmares, and upon waking up in the morning, a feeling of not being refreshed, having an upset stomach and loss of appetite at breakfast time. People who eat their final meal for the day well ahead of bedtime, have enough time to properly digest their food. The result is a much better undisturbed sleep. I find that sometimes, when I feel hungry before going to bed, if I give into the feeling, it causes me to suffer the ill effects of retiring to bed for the night with a full stomach. So now, I try not to eat or drink anything before going to sleep, and that includes water. After disposing of one meal, the digestive organs need to rest between three to five hours before the next meal.

Building Up Good Health Habits

Digestion begins in the mouth, therefore chew properly. An adequate daily bowel movement is recommended since a lack of it is where the greatest share of diseases may spring forth from. Don't become septic. If you have been constipated, and are suffering as a result, you need a thorough cleansing. This can be done simply by swallowing a tablespoon of olive oil along with drinking a large hot cup of ginger or lemon tea without sweeteners in it. Repeating this process every twelve hours until the desired result is realized is undeniably a good idea. And even then, continue drinking a hot herbal tea in the morning before breakfast and again at night before going to bed. Repeat this regimen daily, so that the stomach continues to feel normal, as you persist in achieving the desired health result.

Our bodies must be kept clean. Therefore, take regular showers and baths, and don't neglect to change your clothing, especially underwear. Our body is the temple of the Holy Spirit. "What? know ye not that your body is the temple of the Holy Ghost which is in you, which ye have of God, and ye are not your own? For ye are bought with a price: therefore glorify God in your body, and in your spirit, which are God's,"
1 Corinthians 6:19-20 KJV.

Our houses and areas around the house are to be kept clean, which is not the easiest task. A good suggestion is to break up the housework into sections, taking care of things room by room each day. This makes the task much more manageable. An example of a weekly cleaning schedule can be :-
Monday: bathroom
Tuesday: home office
Wednesday: entryway, staircases, hallways
Thursday: kitchen

Friday: living room and dining room
Saturday night; laundry issues
Sunday: bedrooms.

This is just one example; however, you can fashion your schedule anyway you choose. And since most likely there are males living in the house, they can make their own schedule for keeping up with the yard and surrounding land space.

Have your surroundings attractive and orderly with everything in its place. Pay particular attention to the kitchen and bathroom. These should be the two cleanest rooms in the house; for these are the two places where you put things into your body and throw things out of your body. Cleanliness is next to godliness.

A very simple form of daily exercise can be simply planting a home garden. It will benefit your physique along with other health benefits. Gardening can make you happy and build self-esteem. Some of us were born with a green thumb, and watching our plants grow and produce foods can really boost us with a good feeling. Having a vegetable garden helps to keep money in our pocket as we save at the grocery store. Gardening improves strength as we dig, bend, carry heavy tools, and weed. It is good for the whole family too, as it provides an opportunity for bonding. Besides, being in the sunlight provides vitamin D which especially helps older adults strengthen bones. A broad hat for covering and sunscreen for the skin are not to be forgotten though. And never neglect drinking water while engaging in this outdoor activity, especially on a warmer day.

It is not a good idea to sleep in a room with closed windows. Opening windows at night improves airflow and increases ventilation to the room. This is instrumental in removing carbon-dioxide and inviting more oxygen into your space. If the air outside is polluted, then as much as possible try to change address from living in such a residential area. Cool air can help you breathe better, and if the air coming through the window is dry, then I suggest using a humidifier in the room. One downside to sleeping with open windows if you live in the city can be noise, and if you live in the country, it can be the early morning sound of wildlife, especially birds, which can wake you up too soon. In any instance, sleeping with open windows at night brings with it good benefits, and I encourage it.

A Well-Ordered Living Environment

Like the Garden of Eden, our surroundings should be designed attractively and pleasant, thus resulting in a positive impact on our mood. The best place to live is in an area surrounded by nature. Some folks might only have limited land space with a small yard around the house. Nevertheless, if there is space enough for a lawn, then go ahead and put one in. Plant flowers in the yard too, but if you are not able to do so, then how about a few pots of plants on the porch if you have one, or in the house itself. Bring nature to you. It will lift your mood and brighten your perspective on life.

Houses should have a variety of aromatic smells. For the bathroom, I can appreciate Hawaiian Breeze air freshener. A citrus scented oil freshener can be a nice choice for bedrooms. And for the kitchen, just using trash bags with a lavender and vanilla scent can work wonders for that space. Different scents have different effects, some calming, some energizing. Either way, an air freshener can work to pleasantly change the

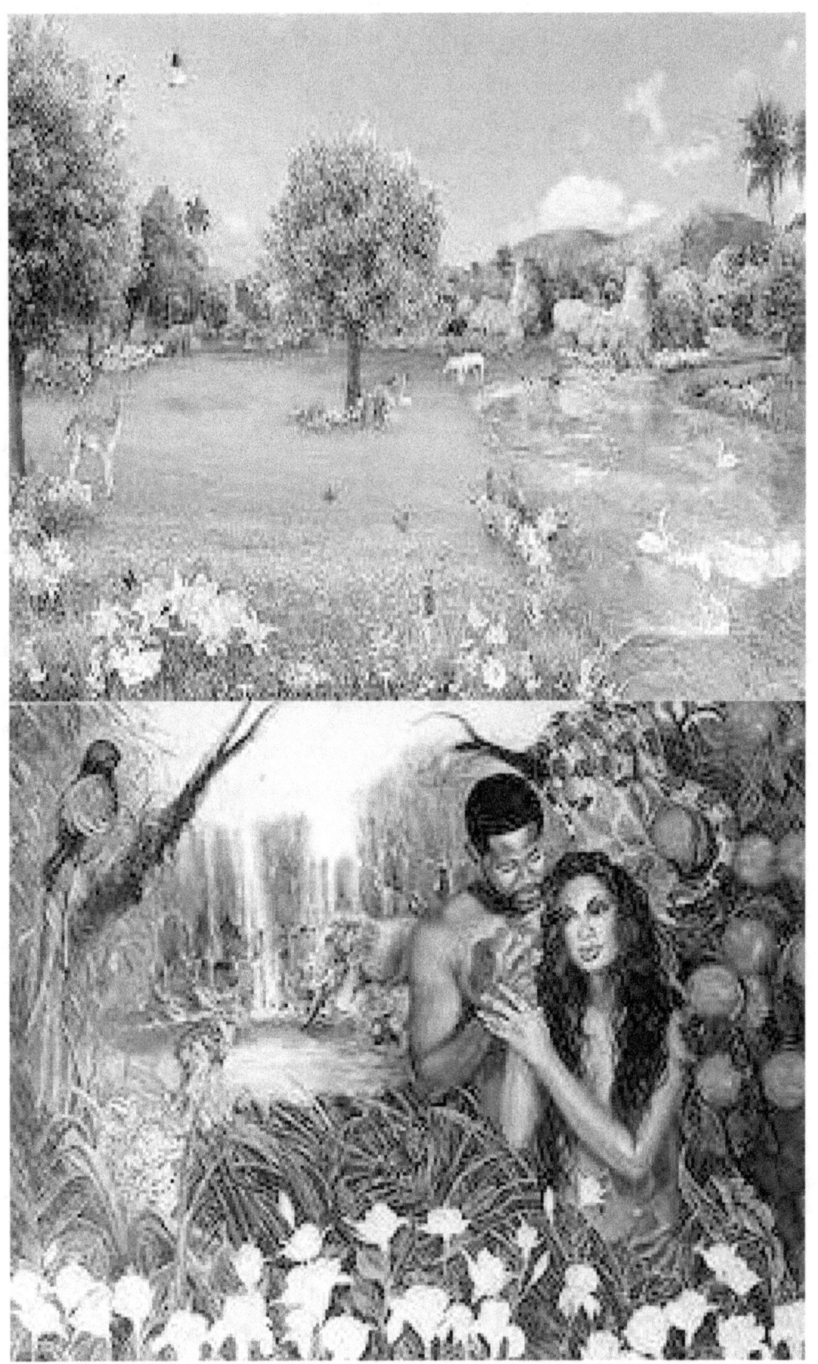

The Garden of Eden

atmosphere in any room.

Consider painting your house. White and pastel shades are very popular since they reflect light, which in turn affects your mood positively. Curtains and blinds in the windows, when pulled up in the day invite light, and when closed at night encourage good sleep. All rooms should have lighting at night, but a dimmer table lamp is what will create a more relaxing ambience for greater comfort.

The spaces in each room should not be cluttered but well organized. The task of cleaning and organization should not be overwhelming if you do just a little at a time.

Some people find that light instrumental hymn music in the background improves concentration and well-being. Others, such as myself, also like the sounds of nature, for instance rain, ocean waves, and the sound of birds.

When the Garden of Eden was created, it was artistically and beautifully designed and dressed. The Most High did this as an example to show us how to keep our own surroundings. Who does not appreciate living in a pleasant environment.

The beauty in nature contributes to achieving both mental health and spiritual wellness, plus a milder countenance. Hence, our own surroundings should also be such as to reflect the original beauty of that garden home, way back out there in Eden.

The Advantages and Disadvantages of Living in the City

There are both advantages and disadvantages to living in the city. I have spent the better part of my life living in the city. And only recently have I moved to a more rural area, where I am once again able to enjoy that which I left behind in my childhood, and in the early part of my teenage years, when I lived in the country.

Living in the city can be stressful although there are some good things about it. However, I believe the bad far outweighs the good. Take for instance people; many people will talk nicely to you, but you don't really know what they are thinking or whether they will hurt you. Deception is everywhere, but more so in the city. There is always much to do and no shortage of employment in the city, but even though there are all types of activities, chances are, based on your temperament, you would have no interest in participating in or attending these worldly activities. You might not care much for the food either, or to become a part of that scene.

A major advantage of being in the city is the availability of transportation and being near the airport. But with what you would spend there on daily transportation, if while living in the country you could save that money, being able to afford to purchase your own vehicle might not be such an impossibility.

There are more job opportunities in the city with higher paying salaries, but the flip side of that is, that it comes with a higher cost of living, a lack of affordable living space, noisiness, and a higher crime rate.

For me, living in the city is like living in an artificial concrete jungle, which cannot be compared to living in the country. Here nature provides an atmosphere that city life cannot provide. Besides, city life has become increasingly evil. That is why we should flee the city. Personally, I opt for the quieter, more relaxed life. I prefer living in the country!

A Schedule for Work and Rest

There are seven days in a week, five of which are working days and the remaining two are rest days. Saturday is the sabbath and Sunday is usually a down day to be enjoyed in the company of friends and family. Under normal circumstances, a workday is eight hours long in a twenty-four-hour period, regardless of the shift. Some people choose to have longer workdays, but overtime in most cases is a personal choice.

The day is divided into four parts morning, afternoon, evening, and night. Each twenty-four-hour section though, is divided into two twelve-hour parts: a day and a night. In the summer season there are more daylight hours in comparison to the winter. Even so, adults need at least between seven and nine hours of sleep per night. While babies, young children, and teens need even more sleep to enable their growth and development.

Circadian rhythm is your sleep-wake pattern over the course of a 24-hour day. It helps control your daily schedule for sleep and wakefulness, and its rhythm is influenced mainly by light and darkness.

GJH 93

Circadian rhythm can be disrupted by various factors such as work and travel among others. This body's internal clock is naturally aligned with a cycle of day and night. And is instrumental in dictating multiple body processes such as body temperature, alertness, sleepiness, and appetite.

In the beginning, the command to work was given in Eden which reads, "And unto Adam he said, Because thou hast hearkened unto the voice of thy wife, and hast eaten of the tree, of which I commanded thee, saying, Thou shalt not eat of it: cursed is the ground for thy sake; in sorrow shalt thou eat of it all the days of thy life; Thorns also and thistles shall it bring forth to thee; and thou shalt eat the herb of the field; In the sweat of thy face shalt thou eat bread, till thou return unto the ground; for out of it wast thou taken: for dust thou art, and unto dust shalt thou return," Genesis 3:17-19 KJV.

Rest is just as important as work and vice versa. Thus, the command as to how we should work was given in the Decalogue which reads, "Six days shalt thou labour, and do all thy work: But the seventh day is the sabbath of the LORD thy

God: in it thou shalt not do any work, thou, nor thy son, nor thy daughter, thy manservant, nor thy maidservant, nor thy cattle, nor thy stranger that is within thy gates: For in six days the LORD made heaven and earth, the sea, and all that in them is, and rested the seventh day: wherefore the LORD blessed the sabbath day, and hallowed it. Exodus 20:9-11 KJV.

Time was also regulated in creation. "And God said, Let there be lights in the firmament of the heaven to divide the day from the night; and let them be for signs, and for seasons, and for days, and years: And let them be for lights in the firmament of the heaven to give light upon the earth: and it was so. And God made two great lights; the greater light to rule the day, and the lesser light to rule the night: he made the stars also. And God set them in the firmament of the heaven to give light upon the earth, And to rule over the day and over the night, and to divide the light from the darkness: and God saw that it was good. And the evening and the morning were the fourth day." Genesis 1:14-19 KJV. Work is important. It helps us to build self-respect. If we don't work, we don't eat. On the other hand, good sleep is essential for maintaining our mental health. There is a schedule for work and a schedule for sleep. It is unnatural to even try to survive on one without the other. Let us therefore appreciate the importance of both and keep the fourth commandment where in lies an overflowing blessing while we enjoy holy rest.

Avoid Harsh Laxatives

It is not good practice to be dependent on laxatives to achieve intestinal cleanness. Although this can help to relieve constipation, overuse can be harmful. Some laxatives can lead to an electrolyte imbalance, especially after prolonged use.

Constipation may involve stools that are difficult to pass because they are hard and dry. However, instead of turning to any form of medicine, a better suggestion would be to take a tablespoon of olive oil, along with a cup of warm prune juice. Such a laxative is also a nourishing food having more desirable outcomes.

A proper diet should correct any case of constipation. Prunes, bananas, apples, and other such fruits, also almond nuts eaten either by themselves, or with oatmeal at breakfast give excellent results. Start with one or two prunes at the beginning of a meal, and from time-to-time drink a cup of hot sugar free lemon tea, or a cup of hot water before breakfast. These are all excellent intestinal cleansers. A well-balanced diet though of 80% bulk vegetables, and 20% grains, will cure constipation and aid in maintaining good health. If unable to have a bowel movement for at least three days it is recommended to see a physician, there may be a complication for which you should seek medical attention.

The Importance of Oxygen

In some instances, one of which is fasting, a person can live for weeks without food, and for days without water, but only a few minutes without oxygen. This chemical makes it possible for the utilization of food. It is an odorless, tasteless, colorless gas slightly heavier than air. Hemoglobin: the most important component of red blood cells is composed of a protein called heme, which carries oxygen in the bloodstream. Oxygen oxidizes other elements yielding heat and energy. Thus, a lack of oxygen in the blood lowers energy, and produces a cold feeling

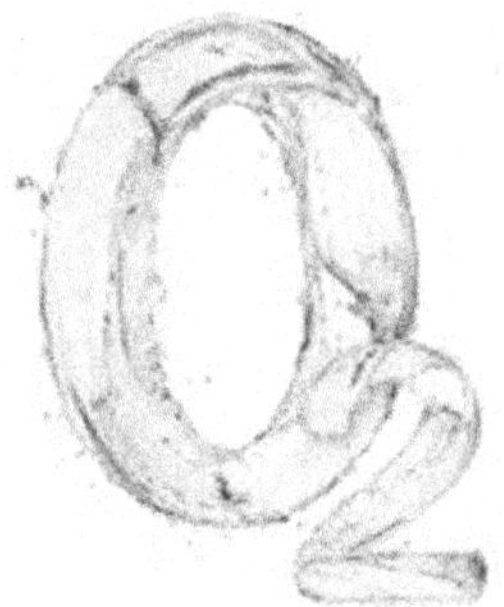

A Critical but Overlooked Nutrient

throughout the body, especially in the extremities. Such a person is said to be anemic. Hence, it is just as important to have an abundant supply of pure oxygen as it is to have an abundant supply of food items in the body. Maybe there are tiny unknown organisms not yet discovered, which are able to live and thrive without oxygen, but most living things including us humans need it to survive. So don't neglect to open your windows, to spend time in the open air, and to breathe deeply. Your body will thank you for the effects it brings in this realm of your well-being.

The Best Drinking Water

To me, water is a mystery. It is colorless, odorless, and tasteless, yet the most satisfying thirst quencher that everyone needs. I learnt in school that it is an inorganic compound with the chemical formula H_2O. This means that it is made up of two parts hydrogen and one part oxygen.

Water is everywhere and in almost every earthly thing. It exists as a gas vapor, as a liquid stream and as solid ice. Now, we all know who made water, but the question is, when was it made. From what I've read in the book of Genesis, KJV, I gather that it was always there in various places. Now let us look at some of these places.

Genesis1: 1, 2 KJV says. "In the beginning God created the heaven and the earth. And the earth was without form, and void; and darkness was upon the face of the deep. And the Spirit of God moved upon the face of the waters." Here the water covered the entire earth, and it could be seen. And on the second day of creation, The Most High "said, Let there be a firmament in the midst of the waters, and let it divide the waters from the waters. And God made the firmament, and divided the waters which were under the firmament from the waters which were above the firmament: and it was so. And God called the firmament Heaven," Genesis 1:6-8 KJV. On the third day, first He "gathered together the waters under the Heavens into one place, and let the dry land appear: and it was so. And God called the dry land Earth; and the gathering together of the waters called he Seas: and God saw that it was good." Genesis 1: 9-10 KJV.

There were also fountains under the earth which brought forth water for the flood, for then, "All the fountains of the great deep were broken up," Genesis 7:11 KJV. Not only that, "But there went up a mist from the earth, and watered the whole face of the ground, And a river went out of Eden to water the garden; and from thence it was parted, and became into four heads," Genesis 2:6,10 KJV. Here we see the creation of various water sources, including wells· "And Isaac digged again the wells of water, which they had digged in the days of Abraham his father; for the Philistines had stopped them after the death of Abraham: and he called their names after the names by which his father had called them," Genesis 26:18 KJV.

The source however that was most preferred by the Most High for man to drink from, was that of the spring. "And Moses lifted up his hand, and with his rod he smote the rock twice: and the water came out abundantly, and the

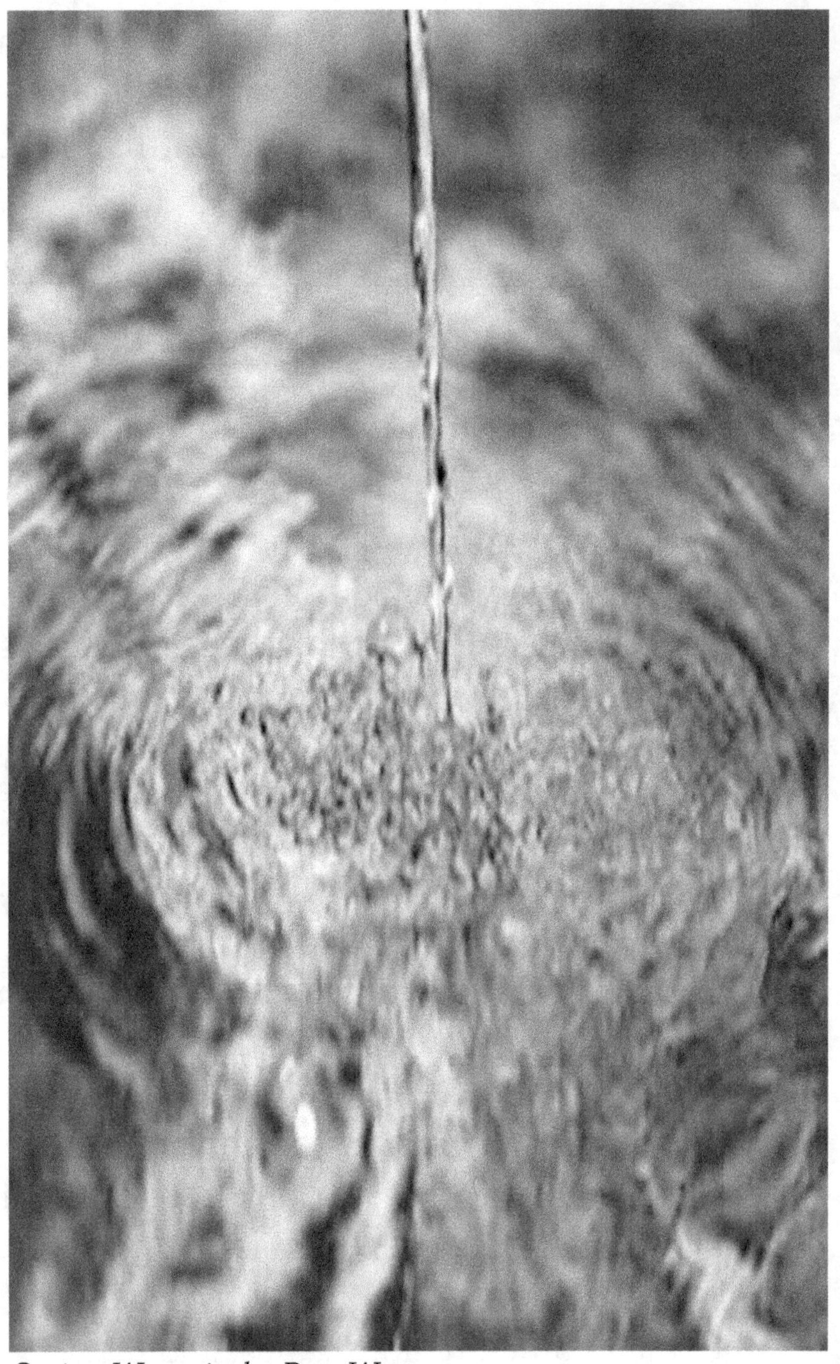

Spring Water is the Best Water.

GJH 101

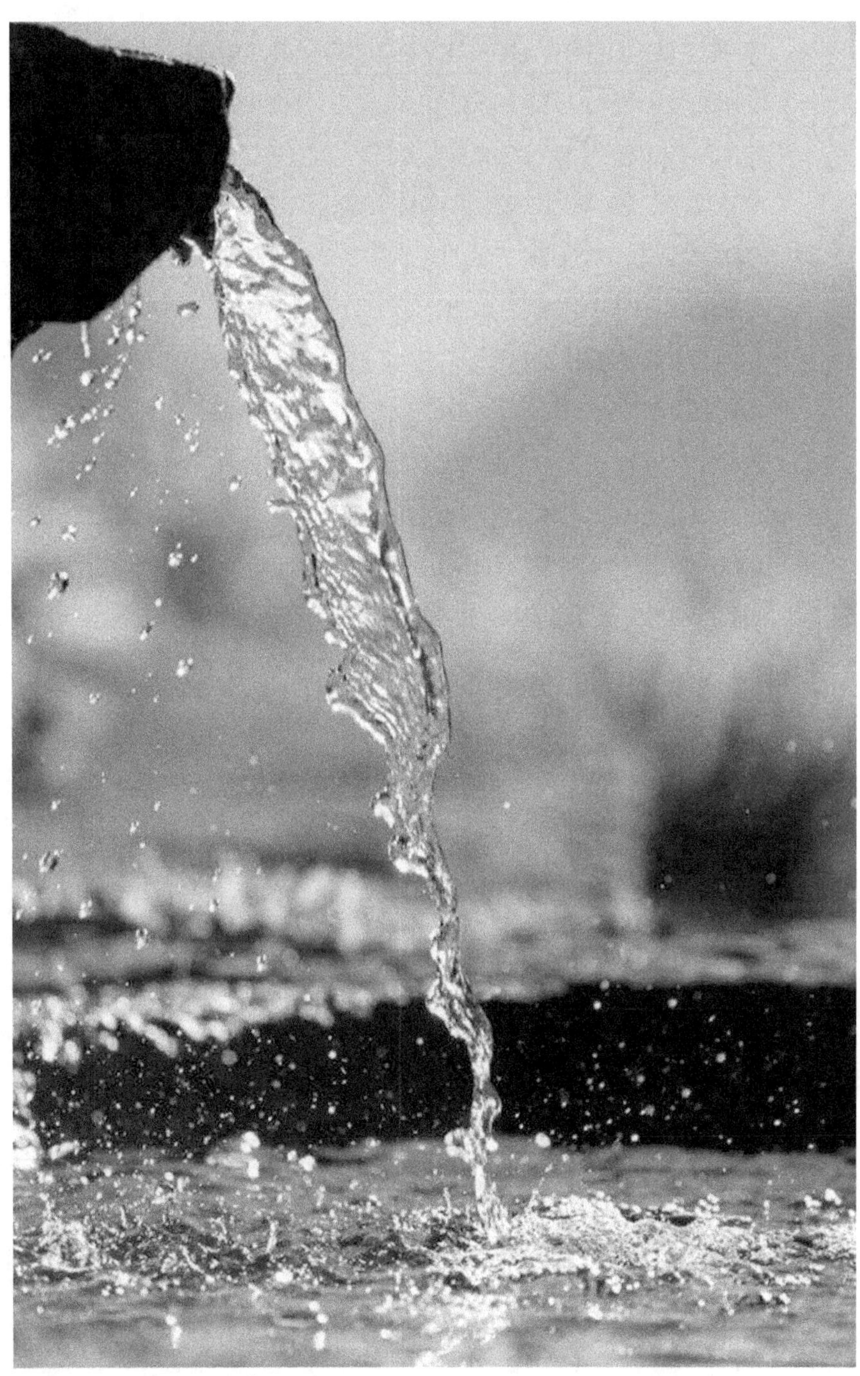

Spring Water is the Best Water.

congregation drank, and their beasts also."
Numbers 20:11 KJV. And this is only one
example. There are also quite a few other
instances where Yahuveh gave His people a
spring to drink from, some even in the most
unlikely places. Plainly then, spring water is the
best natural drinking water. It is alive, much unlike
distilled water, which is robbed of all its minerals,
and is dead. The human body is made up of
about 60% water, and since all body processes
are carried forward by water, then we should be
drinking, preferably the best water which sprouts
from a spring. This water gem is rich
in magnesium, potassium, calcium, sodium, and
other trace minerals. It is alkaline, thus creating an
environment in the body that is less vulnerable to
the buildup of diseases.

Contaminated water is one of the most common
transmitters of typhoid fever and cholera,
therefore, in places where the water is not pure,
two of the simplest ways to purify water in the
home is by boiling and filtration. My personal all-
time favorite water is, you guessed it, Spring
Water!

GJH 103

The Importance of Sleep

Sleep is extremely important to function well daily. Everyone needs adequate sleep which varies based on age. Infants need the most sleep. This includes naps and adults need the least sleep. The time we spend sleeping has to do with the different stages of growth and development. Hence, we must understand what can happen to us if we are deprived of sleep.

Sleep improves both physical and mental health. These stages include REM (Rapid Eye Movement) and Non-REM (Non-Rapid Eye Movement) sleep. Enough sleep or lack of it affects both your physical and mental health. It also gives the body a chance to rest and restore energy. Brain chemicals are very involved in our sleep cycle.

Neurons in the brainstem (where the brain and spinal cord meet) produce neurotransmitters called serotonin and norepinephrine. These chemicals keep our brain active when we're awake. Neurons located at the base of the brain are responsible for us falling asleep. It seems as if these neurons turn off the signals that keep us awake.

Sleep helps us in many ways. We need it for physical growth, nervous system function affecting our memory, performance, the ability to think clearly and for a longer lifespan. People who do not get enough sleep are at higher risk for developing various health conditions including but not limited to anxiety. So, we can see here that based on scientific research, sleep is very important. We need to sleep at least six to eight hours nightly. A lack of sleep alone may lead to serious illness. Hence, taking a warm bath before retiring to bed at night is probably one of the best ways for reducing tension and for promoting good sleep.

Set Goals and Embrace the Hiccups

Everyone wants to be healthy, but not everyone is willing to take the necessary steps to achieve good health. We get sick and pray for a miracle to feel better and to get well, but maybe do nothing to correct wrong habits. If a person is not following the eight laws of health, yet continues to pray to be well, that person is only wasting their breath. On a whole, people must realize, that praying for health should always be accompanied by keeping the eight laws of health. These requirements must be complied with. A good way to do this would be to set realistic goals. Improving health is a journey, and no single task will be able to accomplish this goal. Taking ownership of your health is the best start to achieving health. Know why you want to be healthy and where you want to go with it. Set a starting point and learn the best practices to help you achieve your vision. Don't wait until the end of the year to make a New Year's resolution. Instead, always have a plan and focus on what you want to achieve. Setting too many goals at any one time is just not realistic. Don't give up. Be prepared to keep pressing on until you reach your goal.

Some people like to make excuses as to why they did not achieve the desired outcome, in the allotted time of when their goal should have been reached. Stop making excuses despite the roadblocks. For instance, I am never too hard on myself. If others don't support me, then so what. Maybe you'll miss a day or two from your routine, and that's okay. The important thing is not just to talk but to do it, and eventually you will reach your goal.

The Function of Food, Ketogenesis and pH

Food is any substance consumed by an organism for nutritional support. Calories, which consist of fats, proteins, and carbohydrates, are the amount of energy released when your body breaks down, digests, and absorbs food. Other important nutrients are vitamins and minerals.

The keto diet is an eating plan focusing on foods that provide a lot of healthy fats, adequate amounts of protein, and very few carbohydrates. The goal is to get more calories from fat than from carbs. This diet does not necessarily have to come from a meat source. There were no meat eaters in the Garden of Eden. Therefore, it is quite possible to eat a good caloric keto diet purely from a plant source.

<u>Fats</u> have the greatest food value of all foods; nearly two and one-half times as great as that of carbohydrates.
Fatty foods include nuts and seeds, almond oil, avocadoes, coconut oil, cottonseed oil, sesame oil, olive oil, peanut butter, and soybean oil.

<u>Proteins</u> furnish material for building, growth, and repairs, while fats and carbohydrates provide heat and energy. Obviously then, those who are already grown up, and who do not exert themselves working, have less of a need to repair cells, and therefore need less proteins than do others. Proteins are nitrogenous foods derived chiefly from: -- peas, grains, soybeans and other beans, and nuts. Though not so easily digested as carbohydrates, these foods furnish energy and build up the body.

<u>Carbohydrate</u> foods are non-nitrogenous foods containing carbon, hydrogen, and oxygen. It acts as an energy source used by the body either in the form of work or heat. When carbohydrates are insufficient, then protein is utilized for energy, but when in excess, then they are stored in the body in the form of fat, a source of emergency energy. Those who live in a warm climate, and who do not work hard need less carbohydrate foods than do others.

Carbohydrates can be found in vegetables and fruits containing either starch or sugar. Those which produce the most energy are: - cereals, honey, sugar and potatoes. Excess sugar is stored in the liver as glycogen. Starchy foods require more cooking than other foods, because the starch is surrounded by a covering which cannot be digested when raw. Among others, some principal starchy foods are artichokes, barley, beans, bread, cereals, flour, lentils, peas, potatoes, pumpkin, rice, spaghetti, and whole wheat.

<u>Calories:</u> One gram of fat yields 9.3 calories. One gram of protein yields 4.1 calories. One-gram carbohydrates yields 4.1 calories. The requirements of calories vary with age. According to Forchheimer, the total energy requirement for a man weighing 154 pounds, without any voluntary movement, is from 1450 to 1820 calories. Patients confined to bed, though, are never at absolute rest, except during sleep, and therefore the energy value of their food should not fall below this minimum, except it be under special conditions and for brief periods.

The approximate daily calories required for man under varying conditions are as follows: --
Very hard muscular work 5500 calories.
Moderate muscular work 3400 calories.
Light to moderate muscular work 3050 calories.
Light muscular sedentary work 2700 calories.
No muscular work 2450 calories.

Entering Wedge Society of America et al. 61 – 62.

A person who is overweight needs to cut down on weight-producing foods, keeping strictly within the limits of his minimum caloric requirements. The person who is underweight needs a well-balanced diet, with full caloric requirements. And the average man at work requires approximately 3000 calories daily. There is, however, a great divergence of opinion among dietitians as to the relative amounts of fats, proteins, and carbohydrates required for a well-balanced diet. Perhaps the individual himself will have to determine this by experience.

<u>Mineral salts</u> include -1 calcium, 2 magnesium, 3 potassium, 4 sodium, 5 phosphates, 6 sulphate, 7 carbonate, 8 chlorides, 9 iron, and 10 iodine.

Manufactured foods are partially robbed of these essential minerals. For instance, this has been when white flour is compared to whole wheat, and white rice to brown rice.

The following foods are valuable sources of calcium, phosphate, sodium, potassium, and iron. They include almonds, milk, barley, beans, bread, wheat, vegetables such as cauliflower among others, dates, figs, lentils, oatmeal, olives, peanuts, peas, raisins, turnips, walnuts and other nuts, bran, fruits, table salt, bread, molasses, beets, cereals, pineapple, soy, lettuce melons radishes tomatoes turnips, and bananas. Where iodine is lacking in the soil, it is also lacking in the water. In such regions, goiter is more prevalent than elsewhere.

<u>Vitamins</u>, though we do not thoroughly understand them, yet it is generally considered that they are to maintain health, and to prevent scurvy, pellagra, beriberi, and other diseases. Vitamins A, D, E and K are fat soluble vitamins.

Vitamin A is soluble in fats, and although weakened by exposure to oxygen, it is not affected by heat. Deficiency of vitamin A causes retarded growth, increased susceptibility to infections, especially of the lungs, nose, and eyes, and an inability to see well at night. The skin appears scaly and the hair dry. The average daily requirement of vitamin A is about 7000 units.

The following list indicates the best sources of vitamin A: --Spinach, carrots, cheese, leafy lettuce, butter squash, apricots, artichokes, asparagus, avocados, bananas, beans, beets, blackberries, broccoli, brussels sprouts, cantaloupes, celery, corn, dandelion, dates, escarole, green beans, kale, oranges, parsley, peaches, peas, pineapple, prunes, sweet potatoes, tomatoes, turnip, and water cress.

Vitamin D is obtained from the sun. Its deficiency causes rickets, weak teeth, bowlegs, abdominal protrusion, and weakness. In climates and countries when there is too little sun, viosterol: a fat-soluble vitamin source that prevents rickets, is recommended. Sunlight is also extremely important in the growth, development, and overall health of babies and infants.

Vitamin E is the anti-sterility vitamin. It is soluble in oil and is not affected by heating or cooking. Deficiency of this vitamin causes miscarriages and sterility. An ordinary diet supplies all the vitamin E needed. The best sources of vitamin E are cottonseed oil, wheat germ oil, rice germ oil, whole grain, cereals, leafy vegetables, oats, corn, and peas.

Vitamin K is needed for blood coagulation forming prothrombin, which controls the binding of calcium in bones and other tissues, and also for preventing hemorrhage in newborns.
It is found in spinach and other leafy vegetables, alfalfa, tomatoes, cereals, cabbage, soybean oil

and cereals.

Water Soluble Vitamins include but are not limited to B and C vitamins.

Vitamin B complex is compounded of vitamin B1 or thiamin, vitamin B2 or riboflavin, and vitamin B6 or nicotinic acid. A lack of these vitamins causes pellagra, beriberi, loss of appetite, sore lips, intestinal indigestion with constipation and retarded growth. Vitamin B1 or thiamin, is an anti-neuritis vitamin. It is weakened by alkalis and heat, and highly recommended for infants and pregnant mothers. Hence it is best obtained from raw foods.

Vitamin B foods include --Vegetables, grain, nuts, wheat germ, and brewer's yeast.

Vitamin C (Ascorbic acid) is found in fruits, mainly in citrus fruits and vegetables. Vitamin C deficiency causes scurvy, sore and bleeding gums, sore and swollen joints, and a tendency to hemorrhage.

Vitamin C foods include Citrus (oranges, kiwi, lemon, grapefruit), Bell peppers, Strawberries, Tomatoes, Cruciferous vegetables (broccoli,

Brussels sprouts, cabbage, cauliflower), and White potatoes.

pH: -Our blood is slightly alkaline, with a pH between 7.1 and 7.45. Your stomach is very acidic, with a pH of 3.5 or below, so it can break down food. And your urine changes, depending on what you eat -- that's how your body keeps the pH level in your blood steady. Regular pH levels in your body are **Acidic:** 0.0–6.9; **Neutral:** 7.0; and **Alkaline/basic:** 7.1–7.45. By choosing more alkaline foods, you should be able to "alkalize" your body and improve your health. Certain food groups are considered either acidic, neutral, or alkaline.

Alkaline: fruits, nuts, legumes, and vegetables.
Acidic: meat, poultry, fish, dairy, eggs, grains, and alcohol.
Neutral: natural fats, starches, and sugars.

80% of the diet should be alkalinizing, 20% of the diet should be acid forming, and for the perfect balance in body chemistry, neutral foods must be included.

Food Preparation

When preparing meals, keeping it simple is key. Whether you do meal planning or impromptu cooking, there is no correct method to follow. Whatever is done in this area of daily activities might depend on your own personal schedule. And a good idea would be to discuss with your family what types of foods and favorite meals they like to eat.

One thing in grocery shopping though, is to pay particular attention not to purchase vegetables sprayed with insecticide. If possible, plant your own vegetable garden. It is safer and provides a better variety of fresh veggies where minerals and vitamins are preserved.

Whenever possible, cook fruits and vegetables with the skins. If you must peel them, do it after cooking. Never throw away the water in which vegetables are cooked. Rather, instead of purchasing vegetable stock, make use of this water in gravies, soups, or stews. Do not chop, crush, or peel fresh vegetables or fruits before you are ready to serve them.

Learn to cook well. There is no reason to stay

hungry if there isn't another person around to prepare a meal for you to eat. If you have two hands and a healthy brain, you are not helpless.

Keep your pantry stocked so that there is always food in the house in case of an emergency. Avoid the use of white sugar and commercial sweeteners. Use raw sugar and natural sweeteners instead. Make friends and always try to be cheerful and calm.

Remember that "a merry heart doeth good like a medicine: but a broken spirit drieth the bones," Proverbs. 17:22 KJV. On the other hand, fears, rage, great burdens, and anxieties increase the volume of gastric secretion, thus causing a buildup of stomach acid resulting in gastric ulcers. And now that "ye know these things happy are ye if ye do them." John 13:17 KJV.

"*A merry heart doeth good like a medicine…….*"

Proverbs 17:22 KJV.

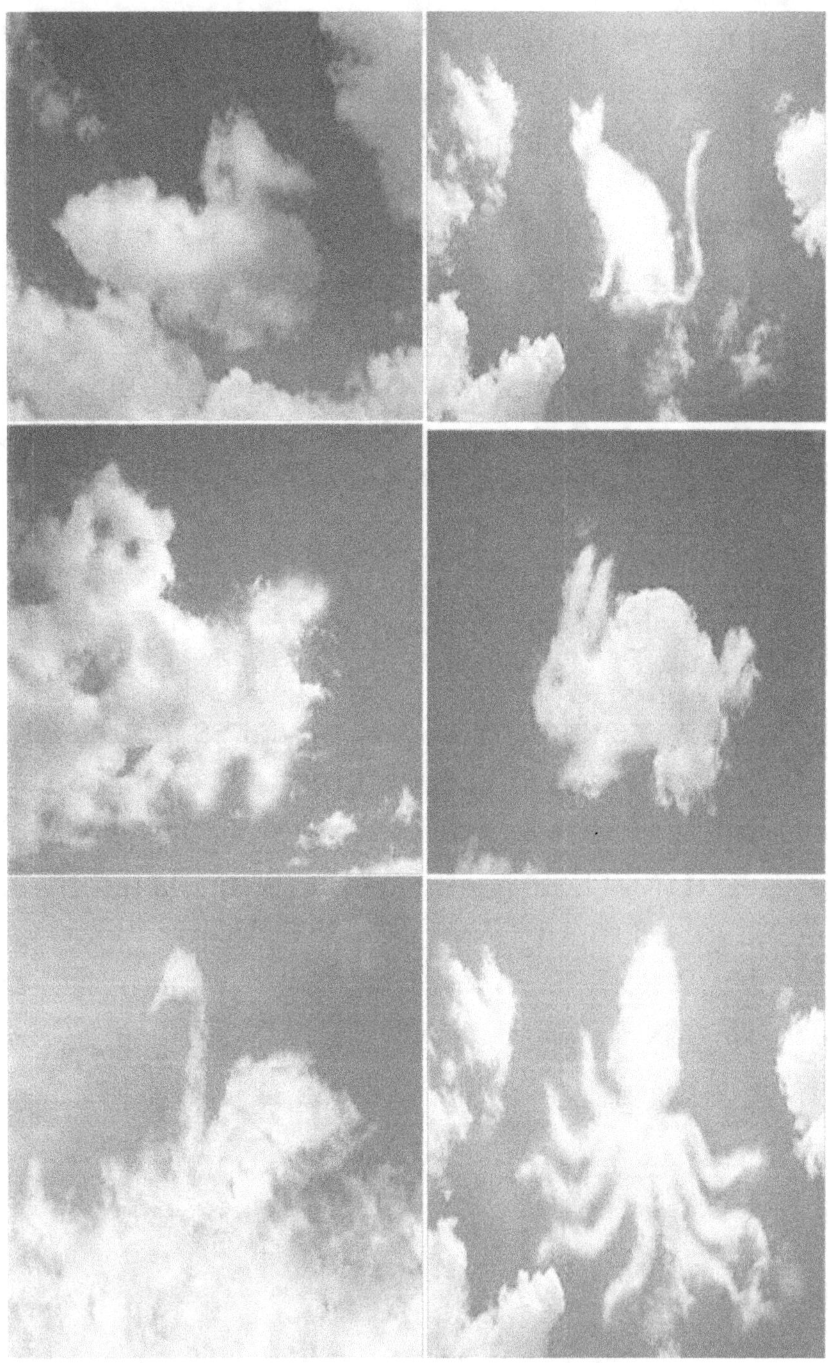

Calming Moving Clouds Movie

GJH 117

And now, as I look back at life while living on the island, I remember how easy it was to be calm, when all I had to do for starters was to look up at the sky above. For there was always a movie of moving clouds, forming animals ever changing, which was more than enough to keep me serene, contented, and happy morning and evening.

PART FIVE::: My Affected Health
How I Became Sick

It doesn't take much to become ill. All you have to do is make a few mistakes which can be fatal. In my case the sickness was progressive. It all started when I migrated from the Caribbean to live in another country having four seasons; a climate that I knew absolutely nothing about. When I first moved there, it was very hot and humid, so I thought that this was the norm. The reason for my thinking was because hot weather was all I knew. I enjoyed being in a new country, going to different places and lavishly spending my money, when a family member said to me, "I notice that you are spending up your money, but

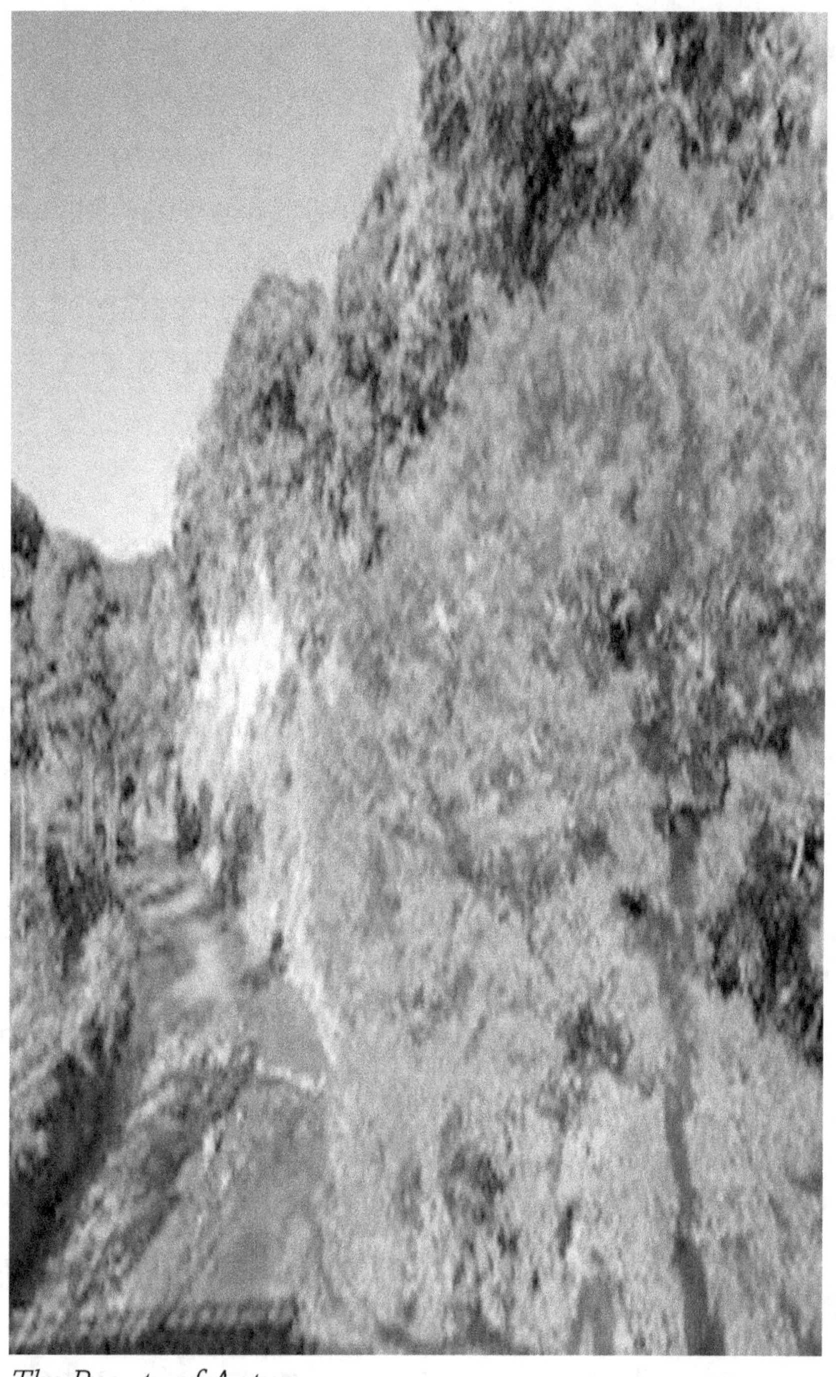

The Beauty of Autumn

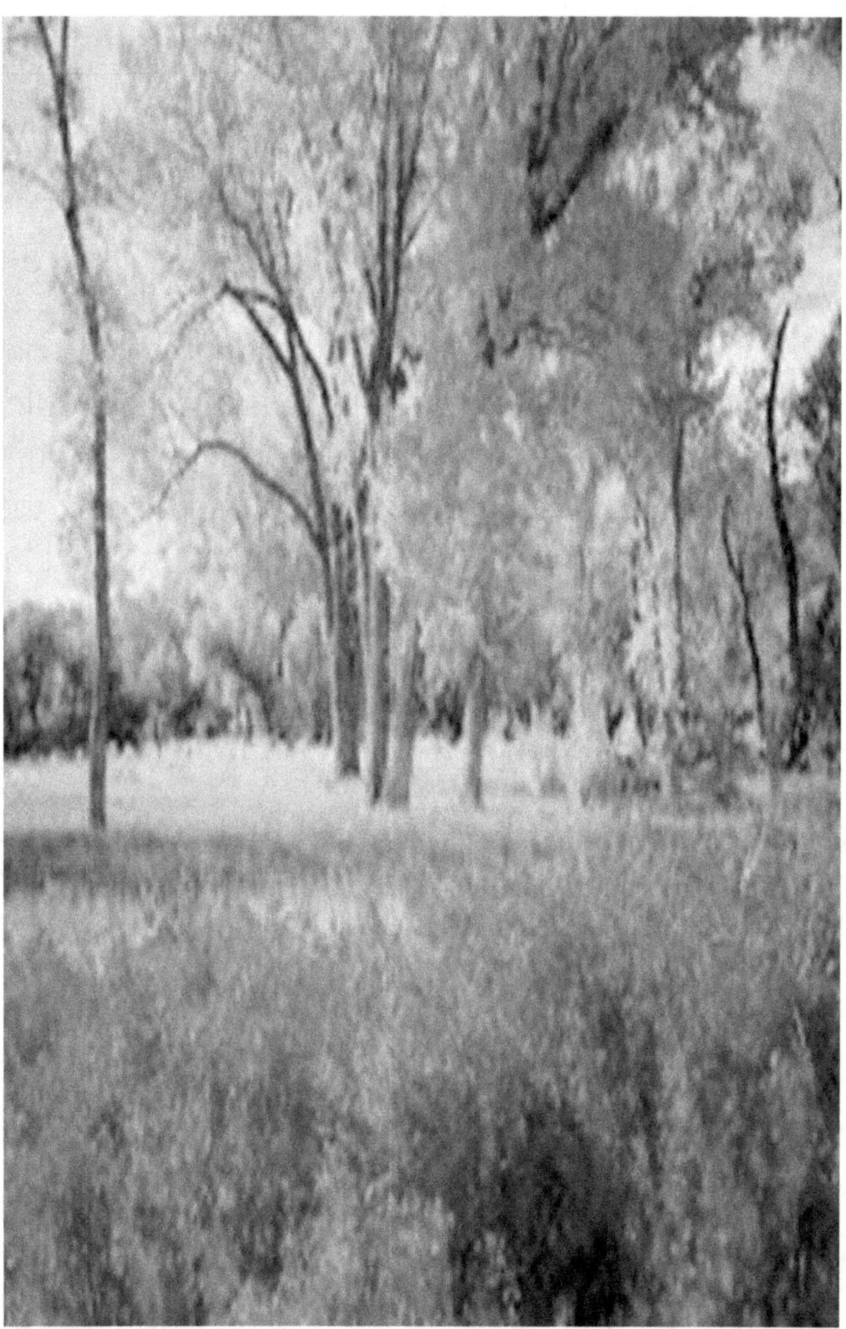

The Beauty of Autumn

you will need some of it to buy yourself a coat, since it will soon be winter." My response to that was, "Oh, it's so hot, I don't need a coat." I was in denial, not acknowledging that the weather would indeed change. I had never experienced winter, therefore, I didn't know what it was like. But the atmosphere soon began to change. Some days would be cooler, and one or two days would be hot. Then I would hear people remark, "Oh, it's Indian Summer." "Indian Summer, what's that?" I asked. And it was explained, but I was still in denial.

The leaves on the trees began to change color. It was no longer hot, but I kept wearing the same summer clothes that I brought with me from the islands. Every day, it got slightly cooler, and my body began to react to the change in temperature. My bones began to hurt, and this felt strange. Yet somehow, I ignored it not wanting to complain. But a couple family members, watching the situation, took me to a thrift shop and got me a coat and a light jacket for which I was grateful. Then a friend took me to the mall and picked out a thick green jacket that would keep me warm in the winter, and I was all set, at least as far as the weather was concerned. But there were other issues, one of which was stress. The stress of being in an unfamiliar environment, and of being around unconcerned folks, of not being able to get around on my own, and of feeling totally disconnected. Everyone seemed to be handling the weather just fine, but I wasn't. The one thing I loved about winter though, was seeing snow for the first time. I was beside myself screaming, "**It's snowing, this is snow. It's snowing, this is snow**," but once it sunk in, I was able to calm myself down again. What was even more difficult was eventually having to juggle work, school, and family all at the same time. And having to eat processed and canned foods, instead of home-grown and vine ripened foods didn't help either. This was when I could feel my body beginning to break down.

The stress got to an all-time high and I felt as if I wasn't breathing properly. My hair just got brittle and fell out. My feet got swollen to the point where I had to buy shoes two sizes bigger, and my body felt so weak that I could not even cover

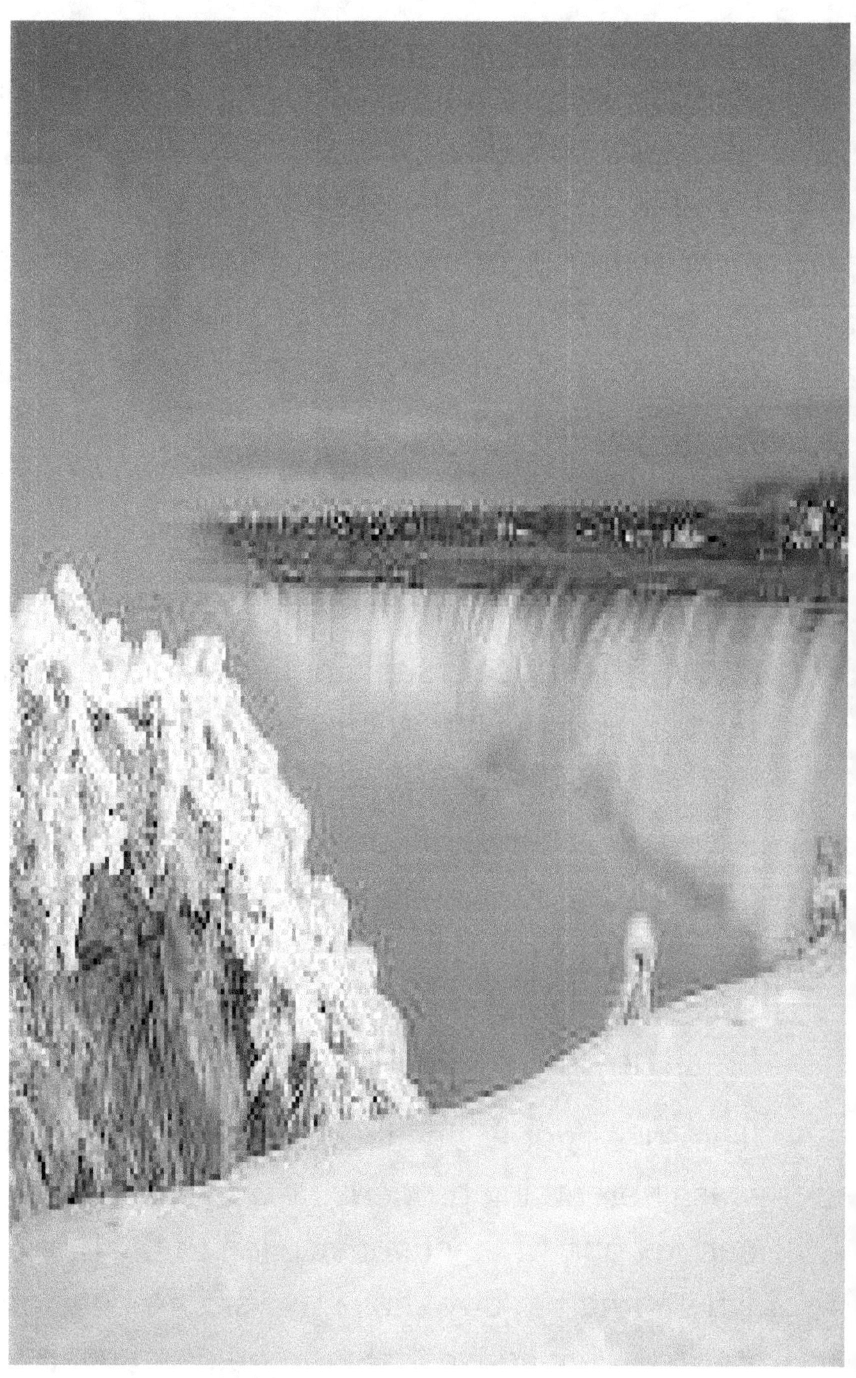

A Winter to Behold

GJH 123

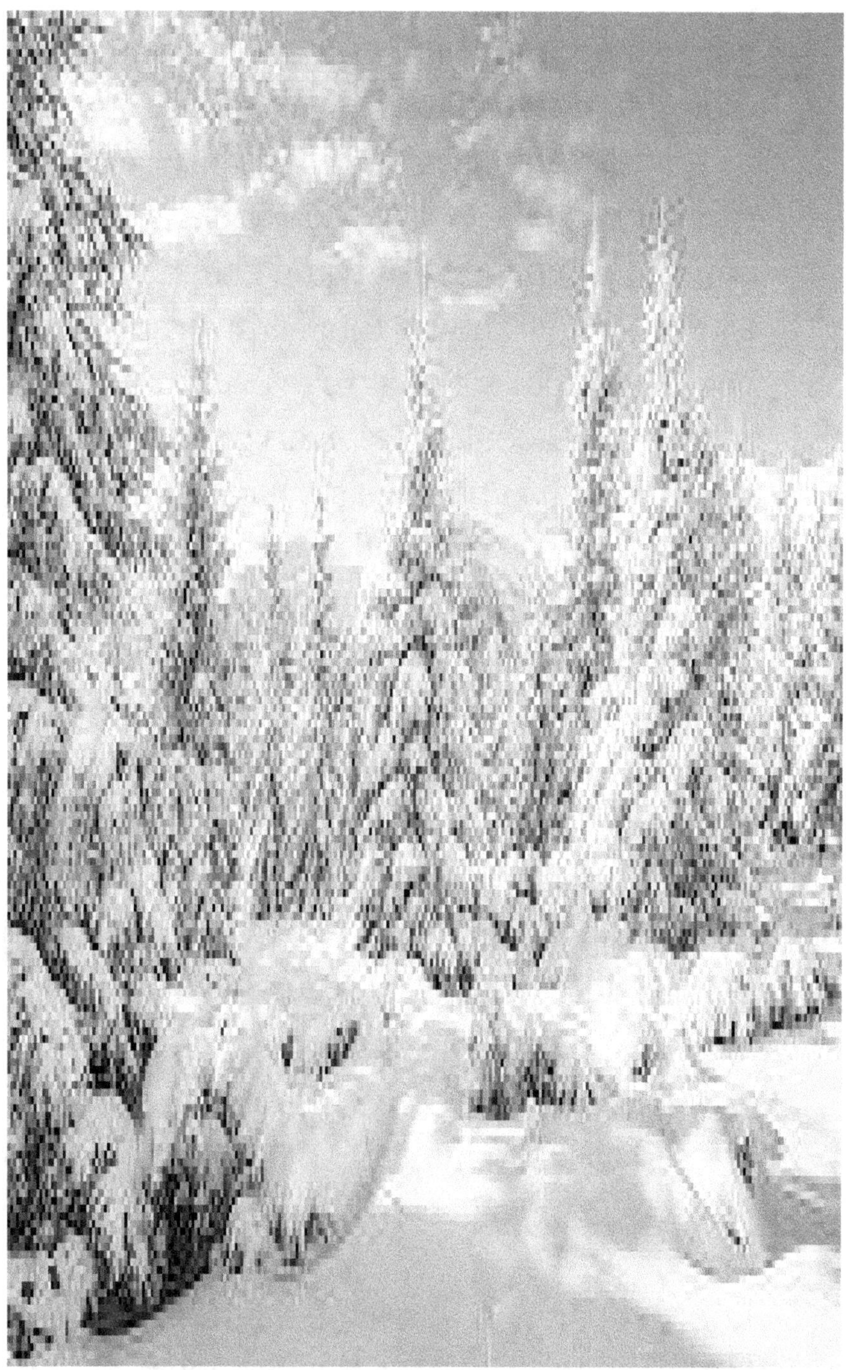

A Winter Wonder Land

my feet. Even if with just a sheet touching my toes, my feet would hurt and burn so much that I had to uncover them. Many nights for different reasons, I would not be able to sleep, and I couldn't sleep in the daytime either. Then my circadian rhythm was totally thrown off. At one point, it was as if I could see everyone, but in a tunnel, and I could hear everyone but in a tunnel. My nerves also became so wacky, causing my stomach to be constantly tied up in a knot. And this by itself affected some very important body processes, which as a result just caused my entire body and its systems to become extremely weakened. Both my hands constantly felt extremely cold, while both my feet felt hot, looking swollen and red. And sometimes, while lying down, the muscles in my calves would just painfully cramp up, and I would also feel arthritic in my legs. This I attributed to the effects of cold weather upon my body. It seemed as if life wanted to leave me, and at this point I decided to begin to fight to get well again.

Looking back on that left behind island life, even the seemingly negative things appeared to be much appreciated then, although at that time supposably out of my reach. Things in nature like the pesty bats, the annoying cockroaches, the ever present May- bees (cockles) in the month of May, the bothersome rats, the playful lizards, those intrusive but beautiful fireflies lighting up the night, little creeping crawling snakes in the grass, biting ants and annoying invasive rainflies during the rainy season, all seemed like something to be much appreciated, now that I felt as if precious life could be leaving me. Such memories, along with all that I felt was good, and together with all that I felt was bad, before leaving that beautiful island life, were now worth living for; worth fighting for, as I would try to hold onto life, just to see and enjoy these things one more time.

How I Regained my Health

I was at home one night when suddenly, something within me said, "boil some water, squeeze a lemon in a cup of hot water and drink it." I then got up, went to the kitchen and did just that. Almost immediately after doing this, I began to crave the same, so I continued to drink cup after cup until the craving was satisfied. Sure enough, I began feeling a change in my body, a change for the better. And from then on, I began seeping the skins of different fruits, but mainly citrus fruits. Added to this, I would liquify aloe vera gel with orange juice, and drink it. Slowly my health began to change. Certain body systems began to work better. My insides began to clean itself out, and gradually I felt life coming back into me again. Blood flow improved. It felt electric, and my health continued to turn itself around for the better, but that was not all.

A Friend in Need is a Friend Indeed

I was relaxing at home one afternoon when a friend called me and told me that a visiting speaker was coming to one of our churches, to hold meetings for one week. I asked what topic he was speaking on and was told that the topic was "The Sanctuary Service in Heaven." Truth be told, I didn't necessarily want to attend, but since she took the time to call and tell me about it, I showed up with my children. And after the first night, I was hooked. I never missed a night. I began to be much more aware of the connection between everyday life and my walk with the Most High.

I was so very impressed with what I was learning, basically acquiring knowledge that the sanctuary service was related to my dietary intake. I learned that when I first came to Yahuveh, it was an outer court experience, where I could eat from all five food groups; but as I move closer to Him, flesh foods should no longer be a part of my diet. Once in the Holy Place, the diet changes from a flesh-eating diet to a vegetarian diet, thus eating from only four food groups, namely fruits, nuts, grains, and vegetables. But it could also include milk, eggs, and butter. The closest walk with the Most High however, was to include a most exclusive diet, eating only from three food groups, namely fruits, nuts, and grains: the same diet provided for the couple in the Garden of Eden. The speaker did make it clear though, that no one could tell anyone else when to become a vegan. Taking that step to dwell in the Holy of Holies eating an Edenic diet, was to be a personal walk between that person and the Almighty; and He alone would give the impression of when to take this step. The teachings at these services were more than I could have expected. And from the first night after attending that meeting, I did not neglect to change my diet to a vegetarian diet and gladly continued from that point on to do all that I could to improve my overall health, and to move from being a vegetarian to becoming a vegan.

The Simplicity of it All

But taking care of yourself and staying fit can be very simple. All you have to do is to apply this uncomplicated strategy. The acronym is

NEWSTART!

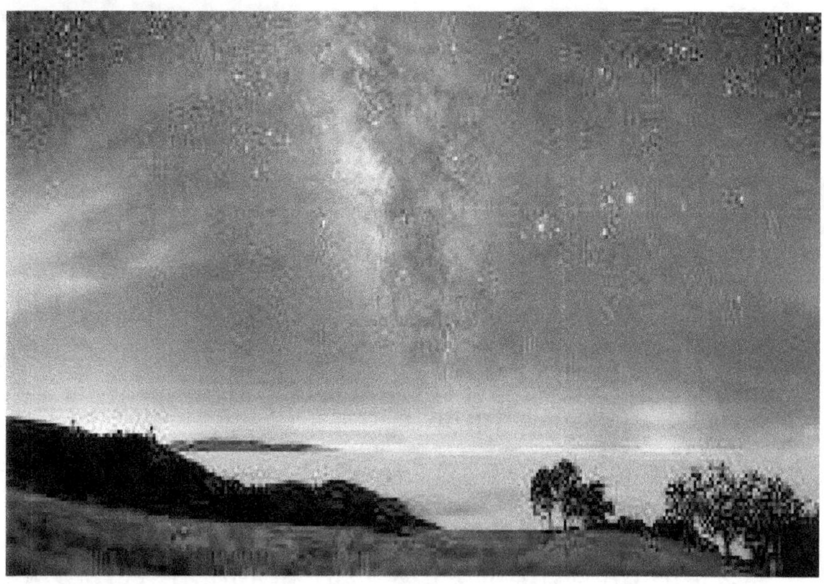

You Can Actually Turn Your Health Around for the Better.

NEWSTART

Nutrition- As you get closer to the Most High, change your diet to vegetarianism. However, a vegan diet is recommended to walk in holiness with Yahushua. Eat breakfast as a king, lunch as a prince and dinner as a pauper. Better yet, eat only two meals daily: breakfast and dinner.

Exercise- Choose a regimen that suits you best. Walking and simple gardening are two of the best choices.

Water- Six to eight glasses is recommended for good daily hydration.

Sunlight- calms you down and may reduce high blood pressure, kills bacteria, improves immunity, strengthens bones, boost mood, and improves sleep quality.

Temperance- If something is not good for you, don't do it. If it is good for you, do it only in moderation (too much of one thing is good for nothing).

Air- Fresh, well oxygenated air cleans your lungs and increases energy levels, boosts your mood, lowers the heart rate, and improves digestion.

Rest- reduces stress and anxiety, improves mood, decreases blood pressure, and builds a stronger cardiovascular system. It also relieves chronic pain and improves immune health.

Trust in Divine Power- The Most High knows everything better than we do, past, present, and future, therefore, He is worthy of our praise. All things are possible with Him, He knows what He is doing. Trust Him!

CONCLUSION

Prophet, Priest, and King Standing on the Cloud

At first glance, you might be wondering why the heading. Well, simply put, I saved the best for last. Let me tell you what happened when I was about six to seven years old. Remember those open houses that I mentioned earlier? One morning, I was in the family's open house, sitting on the veranda where my grandmother was combing my hair. It was peaceful and quiet when something happened, and this was not a daydream. Suddenly, I felt impressed to look-up, when right in front of me above a tall whistle-pine tree stood Yahushua HaMashiach on a cloud. I

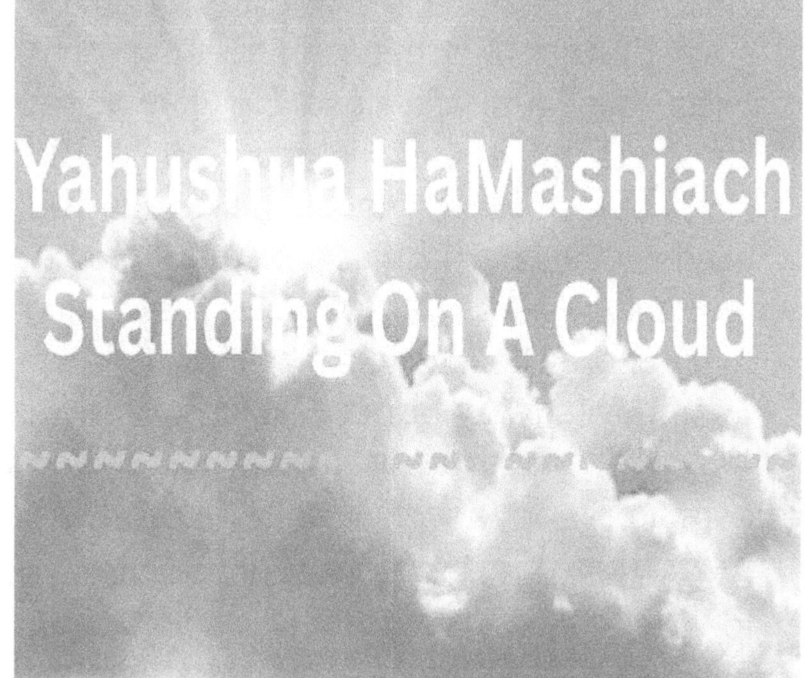

The Majesty of the Son

was a Roman Catholic at the time, but because it was rarely emphasized in that church about Yahushua, I didn't know that it was Him. The person who was glorified in the Catholic church and still is, has always been Mary. They also taught me about various saints, but hardly about Yahushua. Only on occasion, one of which was during Easter, when it was the season for doing the Stations of the Cross, and then He was brought to the forefront. When this happened, I kept looking at the person, and the person kept looking at me, but I said nothing and neither did He. I remember that He was dressed in a white gown down to His feet, but I never saw His feet because it was in the cloud. He wore a golden cummerbund around His waist and His hair fell to His shoulder. He did not appear opaque but was filled with light. That was a manifestation to remember. While looking at Him, the cloud began to lift, more like a helicopter than an airplane. It then moved away from my sight over the roof of the house, and away to the back of the house completely out of my view.

At the time, I really did not know what I was looking at, and I thought it was an angel. Until one day, long after I had migrated to another country, while visiting someone's house, I saw a picture in a magazine having the same depiction, and that is when I realized that the person whom I saw was Yahushua HaMashiach.

While this was happening, I kept very quiet about it, but a few days later I told my family that I saw an angel in the sky. They asked me repeatedly if I was sure I didn't see a cloud in formation, like the clouds illustrated above. But I assured them that it was not. As I look back on that experience, I came to the conclusion that the unrealized peace of Yahuveh was always on that land, and always with us; one that could be felt and seen reflected in various areas of our lives, particularly our well-being. And for this, among other reasons, I praise Him!

All in all, if there is one thing which I can emphatically say I hate, it is that of seeing people sick. I like it better when others are at their best. Sometimes, when folks are suffering, and knowing that this is not what I would want to be experiencing myself, I try to find ways to fix the problem. Sad to say, I am not always successful. But with what little I can do; it always gives me great satisfaction to bring relief to someone who otherwise might not be able to find a solution to their health problem. And this is one of the reasons why I write. Being ill and uncomfortable is no fun. We were meant to feel good in our own skin. So best wishes to all those who read this book. "KETO ISLAND GIRL Living Healthy Being Healthy," and you know what they say,

"Big things: (my God given thoughts and ideas), come in small packages (this book)."

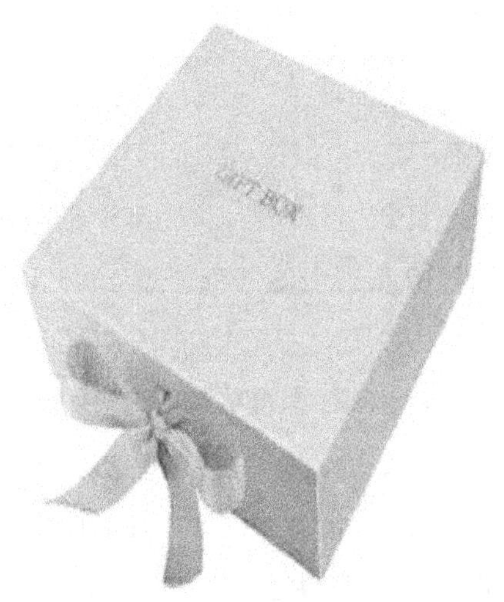

"Big things come in small Packages."

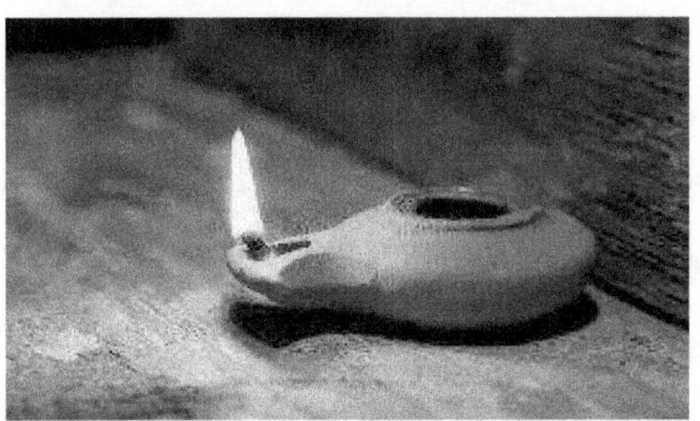

Psalm 23: The Anointing Psalm

[1] The LORD is my shepherd; I shall not want.

[2] He maketh me to lie down in green pastures: he leadeth me beside the still waters.

[3] He restoreth my soul: he leadeth me in the paths of righteousness for his name's sake.

[4] Yea, though I walk through the valley of the shadow of death, I will fear no evil: for thou art with me; thy rod and thy staff they comfort me.

[5] Thou preparest a table before me in the presence of mine enemies: thou anointest my head with oil; my cup runneth over.

[6] Surely goodness and mercy shall follow me all the days of my life: and I will dwell in the house of the LORD for ever.

GJH 137

KETO ISLAND GIRL

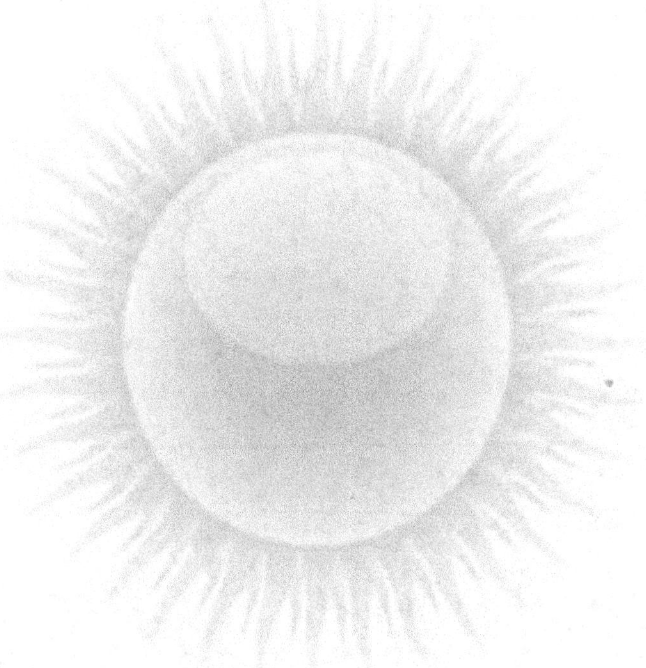

Living Healthy

Being Healthy

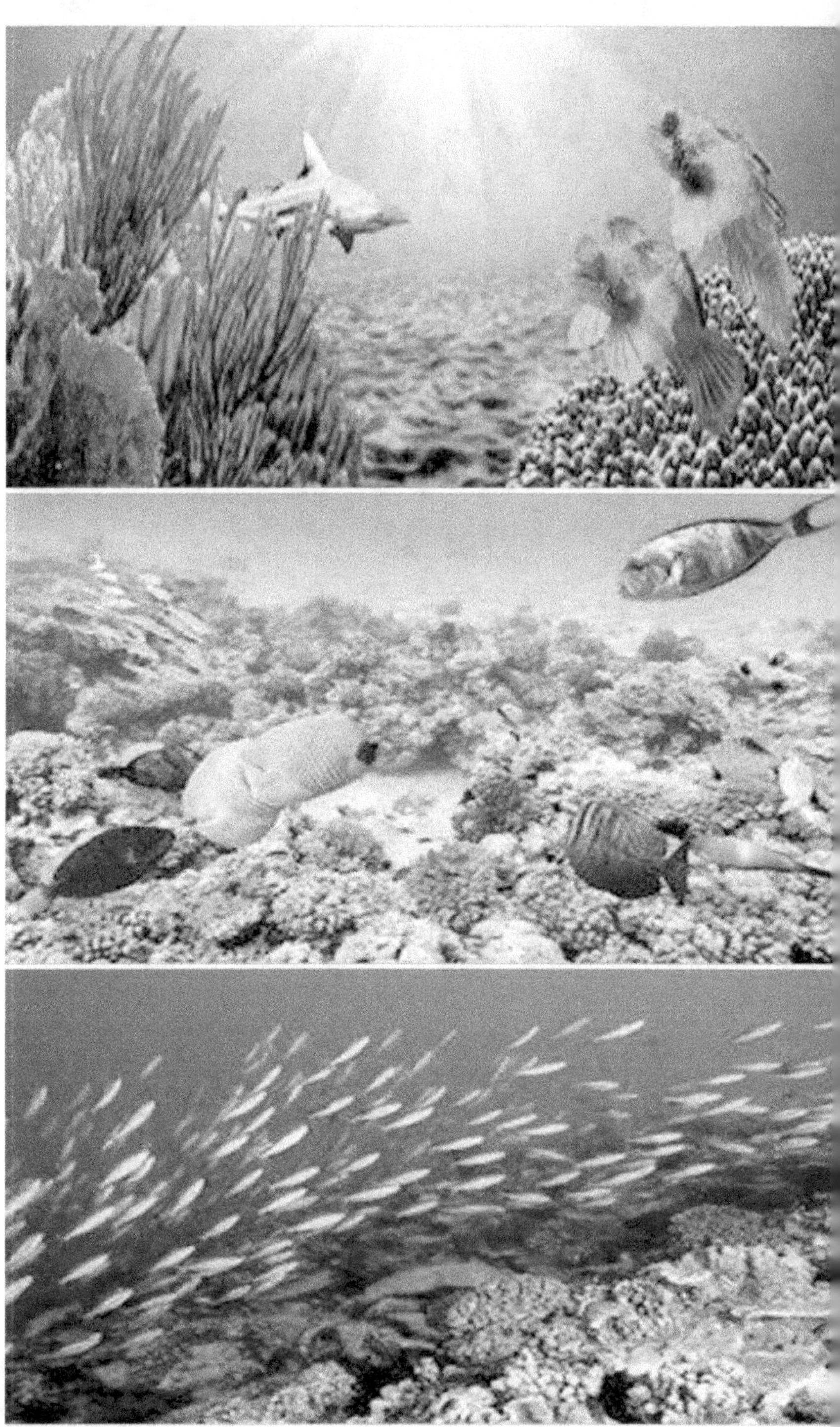

O Island in the Sun

139

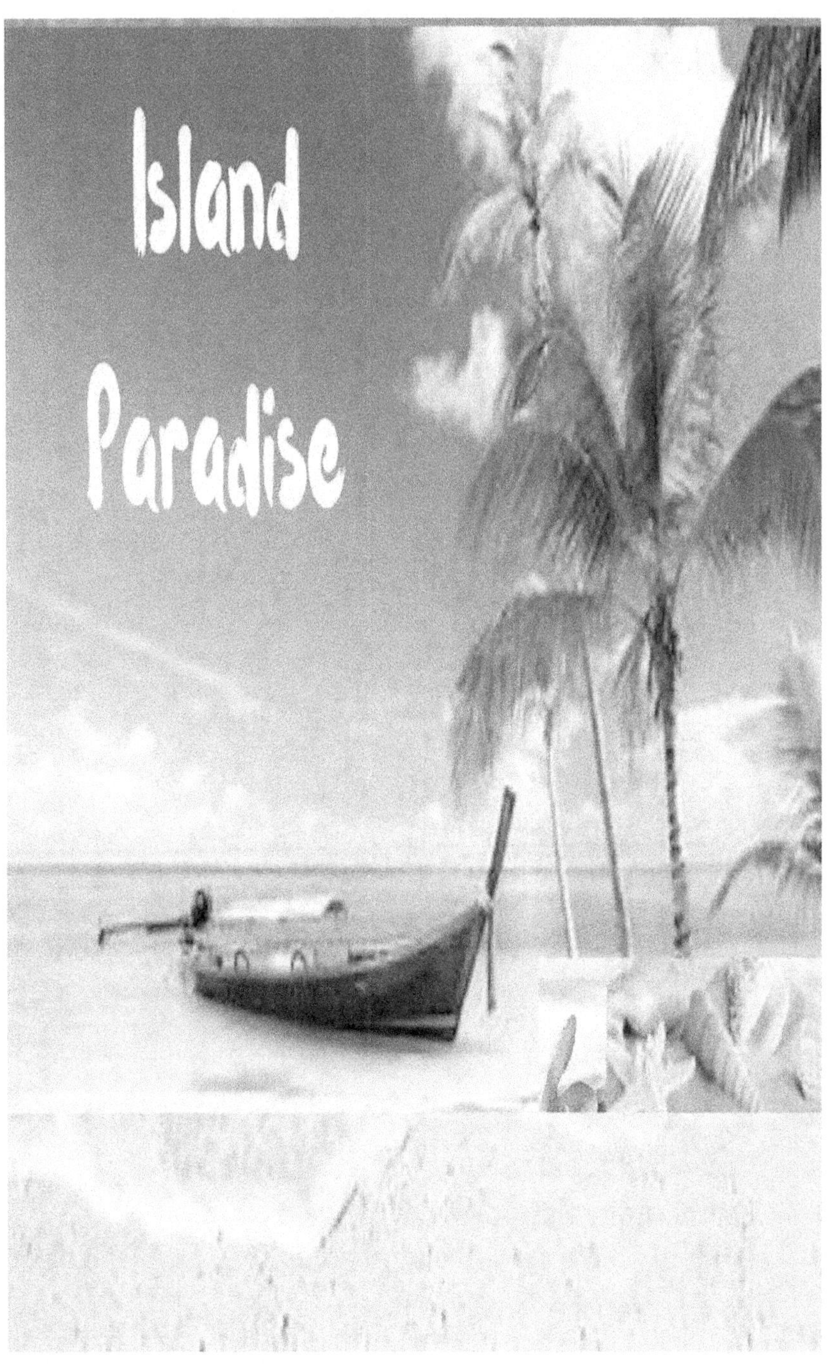

O Island in the Sun

Index

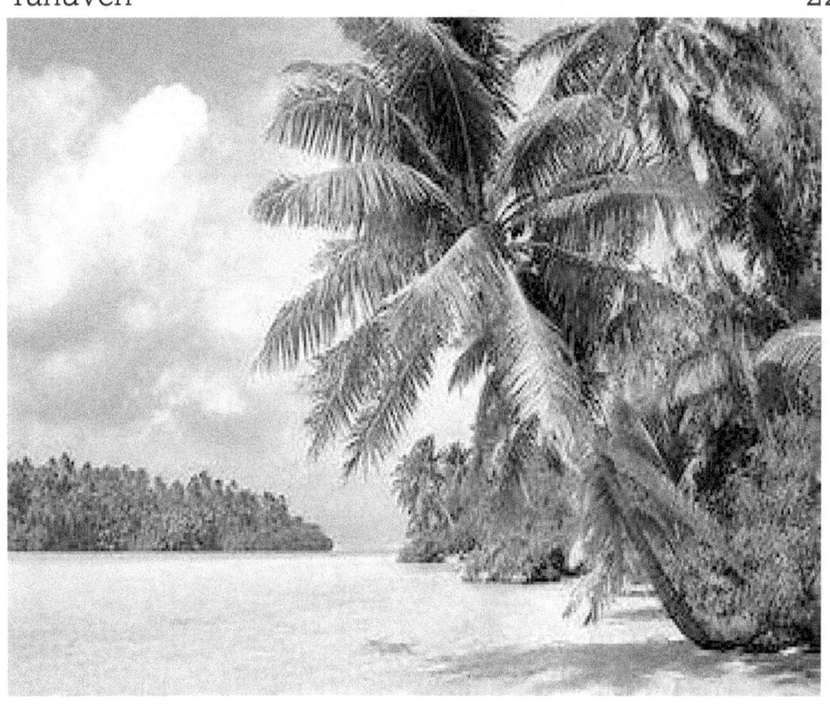

O Island in the Sun

144

www.ingramcontent.com/pod-product-compliance
Lightning Source LLC
Chambersburg PA
CBHW071330150726

47997CB00002B/661